10402

Clinical Radiology for M

CW00967836

Clinical Radiology for Medical Students

Third Edition

G. M. Roberts CBE *MD, FRCP, FRCR, Hon FRACR*
Professor of Medical Imaging and Dean of Medicine
University of Wales College of Medicine, Cardiff

J. P. Hughes *MB BCh, MRCP, FRCR*
Lecturer in Diagnostic Radiology
University of Wales College of Medicine, Cardiff

M. D. Hourihan *MB BCh, FRCR*
Consultant Neuroradiologist
University Hospital of Wales, Cardiff

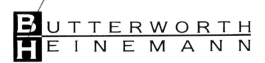
BUTTERWORTH
HEINEMANN

OXFORD   AUCKLAND   BOSTON   JOHANNESBURG   MELBOURNE   NEW DELHI

Butterworth-Heinemann
Linacre House, Jordan Hill, Oxford OX2 8DP
225 Wildwood Avenue, Woburn, MA 01801-2041
A division of Reed Educational and Professional Publishing Ltd

℞ A member of the Reed Elsevier plc group

First published 1982
Second edition 1987
Reprinted 1990, 1993, 1994
Third edition 1998
Reprinted 1999

British Library Cataloguing in Publication Data
A catalogue record for this book is available from the British Library

Library of Congress Cataloguing in Publication Data
A catalogue record for this book is available from the Library of Congress

ISBN 0 7506 1408 0

Typesetting by David Gregson Associates, Beccles, Suffolk
Printed and bound in Great Britain by The Bath Press plc

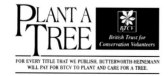

FOR EVERY TITLE THAT WE PUBLISH, BUTTERWORTH-HEINEMANN
WILL PAY FOR BTCV TO PLANT AND CARE FOR A TREE.

Contents

Preface

Diagnostic radiology includes such diverse methods of imaging as plain film radiography, fluoroscopy, ultrasonography, radionuclide imaging, computed tomography and magnetic resonance imaging, and is an integral part of the diagnostic and management process in a large variety of clinical problems.

Partly due to an overcrowded undergraduate curriculum, students in many medical schools have relatively little instruction in diagnostic radiology and therefore tend to be unaware of the value or limitations of radiological investigations.

In this short textbook the radiological appearances of common medical conditions are demonstrated. The new imaging modalities have been included in order to show the role they play in clinical diagnosis and management. We believe that medical students should learn how to apply diagnostic imaging investigations and how to recognise basic radiological signs by the time they graduate and become junior hospital doctors. This basic knowledge will be of assistance in later years when junior hospital doctors specialise in one of a wide variety of clinical specialities, some of which make great demands of radiological departments.

Generations of medical students have helped us in the preparation of this new edition. We have added short sections on how a department of clinical radiology should be used, on minimising radiation doses to patients, on how images are produced, on contrast agents, and on how patients are managed before, during and after radiological investigations.

We also recommend that this book is used in conjunction with the guideline booklet *Making the Best Use of a Department of Clinical Radiology*, published by the Royal College of Radiologists in London.

Acknowledgements

We acknowledge the influence of former authors on the development and success of previous editions of this book: Emeritus Professor K. T. Evans, Dr I. H. Gravelle, Dr Fiona Butler and Dr Tina Hayward. They taught medical students with great enthusiasm, and in so doing illustrated the value of radiological investigations and the most appropriate way of using them for the benefit of patients.

Several of our colleagues have contributed illustrations for this new edition: Drs Colin Evans, Anthony Jones, John Rees, Michael Ruttley, Leslie Williams and Andrew Wood.

Mrs Debbie Roelvink typed the manuscript and Mrs Ros Maylin provided secretarial assistance.

Part 1

Clinical radiology: an introduction

In this textbook students are instructed how to use a department of clinical radiology and how to recognise important radiological signs in certain clinical conditions, particularly those that may present as emergencies. In these urgent situations clinicians may be expected to interpret radiological findings so that the appropriate medical or surgical treatment can be applied.

The introductory sections of the book cover subjects that are important elements of the application of radiological investigations: considering the clinical justification for the investigation, making efforts to minimise radiation dose, and looking after the patient in the radiology department. A basic understanding of the way different images are produced is necessary, and the rationale for selecting an appropriate contrast agent must be understood. Before requesting any radiological investigation it is important to ask three questions:

● is the test really necessary?

● is it likely to affect the management of the patient?
● is it the most appropriate investigation?

The request for a radiological investigation is analogous to a request for a clinical consultation. The radiological report is the end-product of what may have been a long and potentially hazardous investigation. The conclusion expressed in the report is often based on a detailed interpretation process and on a series of deductions based not solely on radiological signs but also on the clinical information, and often on the results of other non-radiological tests.

When planning a series of investigations it should be borne in mind that the diagnosis should be reached by the shortest, safest and cheapest route. The temptation to use investigations simply because they are available and accessible should be resisted.

Whenever guidelines of best practice are available they should be adopted and used.

How to use a department of clinical radiology

Before requesting a radiological investigation the following facts should be borne in mind.

- Ionising radiations (X-rays and gamma rays) are harmful. The effect of non-ionising radiations (such as sound waves, magnetic fields and radio frequencies) are not thought to be harmful at the intensities used in diagnostic tests, but their effects are not completely understood.
- There must be sound clinical justification for requesting a radiological investigation.
- All radiological investigations are carried out in accordance with strict codes of practice conforming with national and international laws and regulations. Radiation doses must be kept as low as reasonably achievable commensurate with a satisfactory and conclusive diagnostic outcome.
- Some investigations cause discomfort; others are invasive and potentially hazardous. The patient's consent is required before some of the more complex tests can be carried out.
- Some investigations require the co-operation of the patient, while others may justify sedation or a general anaesthetic. Some require specific preparation of the patient and others require appropriate aftercare.
- Some investigations cause inconvenience for patients, and occasionally some loss of dignity. Patients are treated with the same care in a department of clinical radiology as they are in hospital wards or clinics.

Radiologists often have prolonged contact with patients and have not become detached or isolated from clinical practice. Patients attending for radiological investigations, especially under emergency conditions, are frequently very unwell and may be elderly and immobile, occasionally requiring resuscitation. Facilities and equipment for these situations are obligatory in radiology departments.

- More than one radiological investigation may be necessary for the complete assessment of certain clinical problems. A logical sequence of tests must be selected on the basis of consultations between clinicians, radiologists, pathologists, anaesthetists and others.

It is important to ask the following questions when requesting a radiological investigation.

1. Is the test necessary? Is it likely to give useful and important information that may affect the management of the patient?
2. Has the investigation been carried out on another occasion recently? If so, why should it be repeated?
3. Are all the previous radiographs and reports available for review?
4. Is the test being requested the most appropriate one? Is there a better or safer alternative?

5. What is the investigation expected to show? 'It might show something interesting' is not sound clinical justification.
6. Is the patient in the best possible condition to undergo the test? If not, what measures may be necessary to allow the investigation to proceed? The radiologist will need to know these details.
7. Does the investigation require the patient's co-operation? Is sedation or anaesthesia necessary?
8. Is there a history of allergy, or of adverse reactions of any sort during previous radiological investigations?
9. Has previous surgery altered the anatomy of the organ or system to be examined? What precisely is expected of the investigation being requested?
10. Are there specific preliminary procedures ('preparation') for the investigation being requested? What is the recommended aftercare, and who is responsible for carrying it out?

Only when *all* these issues have been considered should the request form be completed.

Completing the radiology request form

● Request forms have been designed to give the radiologist all the necessary information to allow the investigation to proceed safely and appropriately. The radiologist is responsible for the safety and wellbeing of the patient in the radiology department and is, in legal terms, 'clinically directing the exposure'.
● Details that may be relevant, especially when the images are being interpreted, include:

  – present or previous occupation;
  – place or country of origin, or recent travel abroad;
  – previous surgical procedures;

  – therapy that may render the patient susceptible to opportunistic infections or drug-induced disorders;
  – previous allergic or hypersensitivity reactions to contrast agents or other pharmacological agents used in radiological investigations.

● The physical condition of the patient is important in determining what radiographic projections and other technical modifications may be necessary. The choice of contrast medium, for instance, may depend on the condition of the patient and on the likely clinical diagnosis in an emergency situation.
● Ionising radiation is potentially harmful. Many radiology departments adopt nationally agreed guidelines of good practice and may decide that a radiological investigation should be avoided during the early stages of pregnancy. Certain tests delivering high doses of radiation to the pelvis (e.g. barium enema, computed tomography of the pelvis) should be avoided if there is any possibility of early pregnancy, unless the benefits of the test far outweigh the potential harm to the fetus. If there is any doubt the radiology department should be consulted. Where early pregnancy is possible the decision to proceed with a radiological investigation delivering a high dose of radiation is a shared decision between the referring clinician and the radiologist who is clinically directing the exposure.

Most hospitals adopt their own style of radiological request form. All have been designed to give the local radiologists the information they need to proceed with an investigation and to arrive at a reasonable and accurate diagnosis. Failure to complete the necessary sections of a request form is inconsiderate and might affect the safety of the patient and the outcome of the investigation.

Clinical justification for a radiological investigation

- All recent national and international recommendations and regulations emphasise that no patient should be exposed to ionising radiation in the absence of a 'valid clinical indication' (*Patient Dose Reduction in Diagnostic Radiology*, National Radiological Protection Board, 1990).
- It is understood and accepted that a 'valid clinical indication' implies that the outcome of the investigation affects or changes the management of the patient, whether by medical, surgical or some other appropriate intervention.
- Every effort must be made to avoid 'routine' examinations because the use of this term suggests that the request for the investigation is not based on the immediate needs of the patient, and that the result is therefore much less likely to affect the management of the patient or the clinical outcome.
- Guidelines of good practice, in terms of requesting the most appropriate radiological investigation in common clinical circumstances, have been published in the form of a pocket booklet by the Royal College of Radiologists in London (*Making the Best Use of a Department of Clinical Radiology: Guidelines for Doctors*, 3rd Edition, 1995). These guidelines are based on the results of published studies and on the collective well-informed opinions and judgements of experienced clinicians, radiologists and others. The guidelines are endorsed by the Department of Health and should be referred to by all those using radiological investigations for the benefit of their patients.

Minimising radiation dose

- There is no known safe radiation dose.
- Man-made radiation accounts for about 13% of the total radiation burden in the UK, but 90% of this is due to diagnostic medical exposures.
- The Ionising Radiations (POPUMET) Regulations of 1988 require all concerned to reduce unnecessary exposure of patients to radiation.
- One important way of reducing radiation dose to patients is to avoid repeating investigations. Clinicians should always ask patients if any investigations have already been carried out. Every effort should be made to retrieve the results of these investigations before embarking on a new series of tests.
- The National Radiological Protection Board's document Dose Reduction in Diagnostic Radiology, 1990, makes several recommendations, including the following:

  - Use tests like ultrasonography or magnetic resonance imaging (MRI), which do not use ionising radiation, where possible and appropriate. If in doubt seek the advice of a radiologist.
  - Make every effort to retrieve old radiographs; this may help the radiologist to limit the number of exposures during subsequent tests.
  - Using the advice of a radiologist, apply radiological tests in the most effective way – sometimes only one investigation may be necessary to reach a diagnosis.

- The term 'effective dose' of radiation is used to give a measure of the dose received by the patient during any particular investigation, and is measured in millisieverts (mSv). A chest radiograph gives a very small dose – about 0.02 mSv for a single posteroanterior radiograph. Using this measure, an examination of the lumbar spine is equivalent to 120 chest radiographs; an abdominal film is equivalent to 75 chest radiographs; barium studies of the alimentary tract are equivalent to between 250 chest radiographs for a barium meal and 450 chest radiographs for a barium enema. A computed tomography (CT) examination of the chest or abdomen is equivalent to about 400 chest radiographs, and a radionuclide study of the skeleton is equivalent to about 190 chest radiographs. Expressed in another way, a chest radiograph is equivalent to 3 days of natural background radiation, a barium meal to 2.5 years, and a barium enema to 4.5 years.
- All clinical staff who clinically or physically direct a radiation exposure, as

defined in the Ionising Radiations Regulations of 1988, require instruction in the basic aspects of radiation protection. Many medical schools in the UK have now incorporated such a course of instruction in their medical undergraduate curriculum.

How images are produced

- Medical students do not need a detailed account of the physical principles of image production but should understand that there is a difference between ionising radiations (X-rays and gamma rays) and non-ionising radiations (those used in ultrasonography and MRI), particularly with regard to their potential to cause physicochemical cellular changes. These cellular changes are produced during exposure and are largely reversible. Radiation protection regulations have been designed to prevent permanent cellular changes that cause long-term complications – a tendency to malignant change (the induction of so-called radiogenic cancers) and a potential for mutations causing hereditary disorders. The existence and nature of the latter is the subject of considerable debate. It is known, however, that the paediatric age group in general is significantly more susceptible to radiation-induced cellular changes and their consequences than are older adults.

- Departments of clinical radiology in most hospitals have a comprehensive range of imaging equipment. They vary in complexity and cost from basic X-ray units that produce 'plain' radiographs to large scanners (e.g. MRI) utilising state-of-the-art computing and requiring purpose-built rooms and special facilities for staff and patients.

- These different technologies produce images in very different ways, ranging from photographic-type film held in cassettes, to fluoroscopy (where the image is displayed on a television screen, having been 'intensified' from an initial image produced on a fluorescent screen), to real-time digital images displayed on visual display units (as in ultrasonography), or digital reconstructed images using detectors instead of screens or films (as in computed tomography). Table A summarises the important uses of these techniques.

- X-rays are generated in specially constructed vacuum tubes; the beam is collimated so that only the part of the body to be examined is exposed to radiation. Other beam limitation devices such as lead shields are added where appropriate. X-rays are absorbed to a variable degree by different body tissues depending on the density of those tissues. The pattern of intensity of the X-ray beam emerging from the patient is reflected in the variable grey shades of the resultant radiograph: black areas indicate areas or structures of low density (e.g. air in lungs), and white areas indicate structures that have a relatively

Table A   Summary of the uses of imaging techniques

Note: Plain film radiography (Fig. A) and contrast studies, with or without fluoroscopy or digital imaging, form the majority of investigations carried out in a general department. This table gives a summary of the uses of alternative or complementary imaging techniques.

Technique	Main indications
Ultrasonography (Fig. B)	Obstetric scanning. Neonatal brain imaging. Urinary tract and abdominal masses in childhood. Abdominal scanning in adults – masses, liver, abscesses, etc. Ocular, thyroid, cardiac and testicular scanning. Control of biopsy and drainage procedures. Duplex scanning of vascular disorders
Computed tomography (CT) (Fig. C)	Intracranial scanning. Chest – lungs, mediastinum. Abdomen – all parts and retroperitoneum. Staging malignant tumours and monitoring treatment. Early assessment of major trauma, especially involving contents of chest and abdomen. Guidance of biopsy and drainage procedures
Radionuclide imaging (Fig. D, E)	Skeleton – infection, early trauma, metastases. Urinary tract – scars, obstruction, function. Cardiac function and ischaemia. Lungs – infarcts. General infection and inflammation – WBC studies. Blood loss – RBC studies. Biliary excretion and leaks
Magnetic resonance imaging (MRI) (Fig. F)	Brain and spine. Joint disorders. Cardiac and vascular diseases. Breasts. Rapidly developing technology subject to evaluation. Expanding role. Definite contraindications – metallic implants, foreign bodies, pacemakers, etc.

WBC, white blood cell; RBC, red blood cell.

high density (e.g. bone). The artificial introduction of high atomic number elements, such as barium or iodine-containing contrast agents, will allow the internal anatomy of otherwise uniform soft-tissue density structures or organs (i.e. grey shades on the radiograph) to be outlined.

- Gamma rays are emitted by certain radioactive isotopes as they decay. This property is used in radionuclide imaging, where isotopes are 'tagged' to compounds that are selectively concentrated or excreted by certain organs. Technetium-99m is the most commonly used isotope in medical diagnosis and has a half-life of only 6 hours, so that much of the radio-activity has decayed within an acceptably short period of time. This reduces the radiation burden to the patient. Gamma radiation is detected over the surface of the body by a specially constructed gamma camera and images are produced which represent the pattern and intensity of radioactivity within an organ or tissue.

- A study carried out recently in the UK showed that many doctors were unaware that CT used X-rays and that MRI did not.

- In computed tomography the X-ray tube revolves around the patient and the emergent beam is picked up by detectors. Images are computerised from multiple measurements of tissue attenuation of the

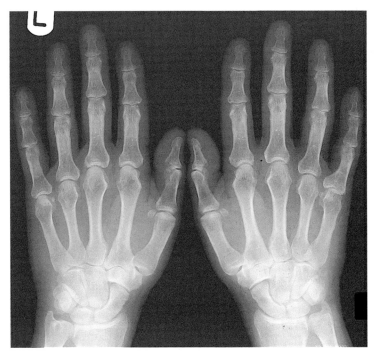

Figure A Plain radiograph of the hands

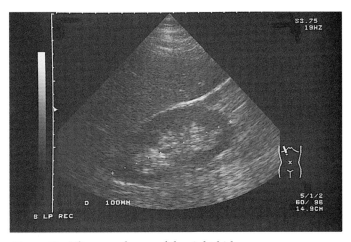

Figure B Ultrasound scan of the right kidney

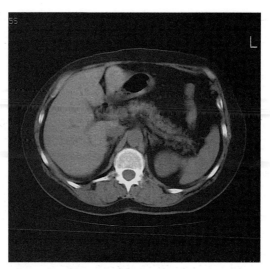

Figure C CT scan of the upper abdomen. The liver, pancreas, spleen, aorta and upper pole of the left kidney are shown

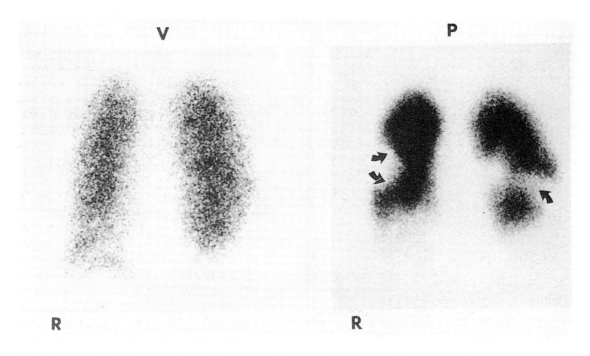

Figure D Isotope lung scan: the ventilation scan V is normal; P, the perfusion scan of the same patient, demonstrates multiple peripheral defects consistent with pulmonary embolism

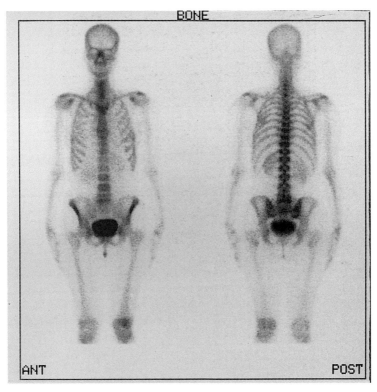

Figure E Normal isotope bone scan

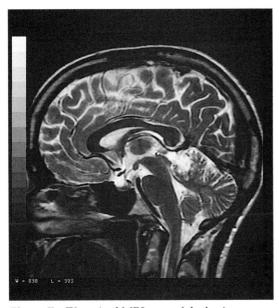

Figure F T2 sagittal MRI scan of the brain

beam during the revolution of the beam around the part of the anatomy being investigated. 'Slices' are obtained at predetermined intervals (i.e. thicknesses). The images produced show cross-sectional slices of the body. In comparison with plain radiographs the visual grey scale is enhanced to improve organ visualisation and definition. The image can also be manipulated to give additional detail about tissues of widely varying density, e.g. bone and soft tissues. Furthermore, these scans provide so much mathematical data that consecutive 'slices' can be reconstructed to give two- or three-dimensional representations of body and organ anatomy. Dense contrast agents can be used to demonstrate the internal anatomy of certain organs, e.g. vascular structures, urinary tract, intestinal tract. Much lower contrast agent densities (concentrations) are necessary for CT, partly because of the enhancement effect of the digital computation techniques used.

- In ultrasonography a transducer is used to produce a high frequency sound which passes through the skin (which is in close contact with the transducer) into the body tissues. The latter may be good or bad conductors of sound – fluid is a good conductor, air is not. The sound waves are reflected at tissue interfaces to produce echoes, which are in turn detected by the transducer and converted into a signal to produce images. Real-time scanning produces moving images (e.g. heart movements in a fetus) and this technique can be refined further by combining real-time sonography with Doppler signals from flowing blood to produce duplex scans for the investigation of the vascular system.

- MRI utilises radio waves to generate signals in a much more complex way than previous imaging techniques. An MRI scanner comprises a large circular magnet that generates magnetic field intensities of between 0.2 and 2.0 tesla for diagnostic purposes. Under the influence of external magnetic forces the hydrogen nuclei of body fluid (water and lipids) behave like small magnets that respond to external radio frequencies under certain conditions by producing their own radio frequencies. These in turn are detected by surface coils and augmented into signals which are strong enough to be converted into images.

- Whereas sonographic images depend on the positioning of the transducer to produce cross-sectional images, in MRI images of parts of the body in several planes can be produced from the signals generated while the patient remains in one position inside the magnet. This is known as the multiplanar capability of MRI and is recognised to be one great advantage of the technique.

Contrast agents used in radiological investigations

- It has been pointed out that most body tissues and organs have very similar densities and therefore attenuate X-rays to an equal extent. Thus the internal structure of many organs is not apparent on plain radiographs, conventional tomography or fluoroscopy.
- Some organs contain air or gas; these have low densities and do not attenuate X-rays, giving normal lungs and certain parts of the intestinal tract their 'blackness'. This is known as negative contrast and is useful in outlining disorders of the lungs (e.g. consolidation) and some diseases of the alimentary tract (e.g. obstruction, perforation).
- Further information is provided by artificially introducing high density contrast agents, containing barium sulphate or iodine salts, into these organs by mouth, by direct infusion or by intravenous or intra-arterial injection.
- The same iodine-containing contrast agents are used in conjunction with CT and for interventional vascular techniques and therapeutic measures such as abscess drainage and relief of obstruction (e.g. in bile ducts) by internal stents.
- Alternative 'contrast' agents are available for use with ultrasonography and with MRI. These are the subject of current evaluation, development and refinement. They will undoubtedly improve the diagnostic value of these techniques in the future.

Barium contrast agents

These are manufactured for use with minimum preparation apart from the addition of water, although there are certain instructions regarding their use that must be adhered to. They are non-sterile and are used in the alimentary tract, usually in conjunction with air insuflation to produce so-called 'double-contrast' examinations. Although barium ions themselves are very toxic, they are not absorbed from these contrast agents. The latter are therefore safe; barium salts have been used for this purpose since 1914. There have been some reports of skin rashes and joint pains following their use, but most of the reported reactions are due to other agents and devices used in barium studies rather than the contrast agents themselves.

Iodinated contrast agents

Apart from one preparation that is used specifically in the alimentary tract, these agents are prepared for use in special sterile containers. They are water-soluble salts and are used to outline the urinary tract and the cardiovascular system in particular.

Iodinated contrast agents vary in their physical properties and in their iodine concentration. They share one major disadvantage – their tendency to produce hypersensitivity reactions, ranging from mild wheezing, skin eruptions and nausea to anaphylactoid reactions and cardiac arrest. Mild reactions are common and efforts have been made over many years to develop safer agents. Currently, non-ionic solutions are used to reduce the frequency of side-effects, particularly in those individuals who may be at some additional risk of a reaction – those with atopic tendencies and asthma in particular.

Prevention of reactions using corticosteroid prophylaxis is a controversial issue and this measure is not universally accepted.

Full resuscitation facilities are required for investigations using iodinated contrast agents, and none of these investigations should be embarked upon where there is no valid clinical justification.

Looking after the patient in the radiology department

- The majority of investigations carried out in a radiology department involve uncomplicated plain radiographs that require virtually no preparation of the patient or post-investigation care; other investigations may be invasive, time consuming, and involve some potential hazard or risk of complications. Here, the department adopts a set of procedures and safeguards that are designed to protect the patient or to minimise the effects of the investigations and to improve the safety margin. At all times the risk of an investigation must be balanced against the likely benefit to the patient – and integral part of the clinical justification process.

- Quite apart from national and local codes of practice in relation to radiation protection, a department of radiology is likely to have written procedures covering the following circumstances:

  - Preparation of patients for a large variety of tests. These include topics such as starvation, antibiotic cover and measures to be used in diabetic patients.
  - Resuscitation techniques following untoward reactions to agents used in certain tests, such as contrast media. These measures are agreed in conjunction with anaesthetists and others who may be expected to attend and give practical advice during these emergencies in a radiology department.
  - Procedures that are necessary following some invasive procedures, especially those involving prolonged vascular investigations and other interventional techniques. Care of wounds, puncture sites, catheters, stents, drainage equipment and infusion catheters fall into this category. If there is a risk of blood loss or loss of other body fluids regular monitoring of patients is necessary. These measures are often instigated by radiologists, who will then share the responsibility for the patient's safety and welfare with the referring clinicians and ward staff. It is particularly important that these procedures and the lines of responsibility are worked out in advance, and that all written instructions are adhered to.
  - Radiology departments will have written procedures for dealing with cross-infections, hepatitis and acquired immune deficiency syndrome (AIDS), for dealing with soiled equipment, for appropriate sterilisation procedures, and for ensuring the cleanliness of radiological equipment used in sterile techniques.

- Recovery facilities are often provided in those departments where patients are likely to be administered general anaesthesia for certain investigations.
- The patient is expected to give informed consent for many of the more complex radiological procedures. Some patient counselling may also be necessary in relation to imaging techniques, e.g. coping with claustrophobia in MRI, or in dealing with complicated obstetric problems following ultrasonographic monitoring of the fetus.
- Radiology departments seek to inform patients about radiological investigations; this information may take the form of suitably prepared letters, information sheets, pamphlets, posters or video films.
- Finally, the aftercare of patients may extend even beyond transportation to patients' homes – this particularly applies to investigations using radionuclides, which may be released from the body over several hours (and which may contaminate clothing), or which may be secreted, for example in breast milk. Written instructions are available to cover all these eventualities.

It is important that all doctors referring patients for radiological procedures are aware of these requirements, familiarise themselves with the key instructions, and ensure that the appropriate aftercare is carried out. Doubts or misunderstandings are best resolved by dialogue; radiologists are available for discussions regarding any of the above procedures and can justify the measures and give advice on their appropriate use.

Part 2

Chapter 1

The chest

Chest radiographs are the most commonly requested radiological investigations, particularly in clinical emergencies. A sound knowledge of the signs of disease and their correct interpretation is essential, especially for junior medical staff dealing with such emergencies.

Correct identification of anatomical structures and a knowledge of their normal varients is vital when examining a chest radiograph. Misinterpretation of an opacity due to a normal structure may lead to serious errors in diagnosis. An opaque lesion on the skin or in the thoracic wall will produce an opacity superimposed on the lungs which may be mistaken for an intrapulmonary lesion. Careful clinical examination will help to avoid such errors.

Chest radiographs are normally obtained in full inspiration, the erect patient facing the X-ray film cassette with the X-ray beam passing in a posteroanterior (PA) direction. Patients who are so ill that they must be examined on the ward or lying supine on a stretcher usually have radiographs of the chest taken anteroposteriorly (AP). It is important to realise that such variations in technique can produce distinctive differences in the radiographs, as shown in Figure 1.1 and summarised in Table 1.1.

Table 1.2 summarises the features of the normal chest radiograph.

Projections used in chest radiography

A PA radiograph obtained in deep inspiration provides most information about the chest, and is the 'gold standard' to aim for. A number of additional projections may be used under certain circumstances (Table 1.3). Any lesion shown on a PA radiograph may be localised or assessed further using additional projections or alternative techniques, e.g. CT.

Pulmonary abnormalities

The patterns of abnormalities shown on a chest radiograph may be broadly classified into:

- unilateral opacification
- large opacities within the lungs
- well-defined rounded opacities
- small opacities up to 5 mm in size
- abnormal linear opacities
- localised areas of increased transradiancy
- large areas of increased transradiancy
- mediastinal abnormalities.

Several of these patterns may coexist, and may be seen in association with abnormalities of the heart and pulmonary vessels, or in

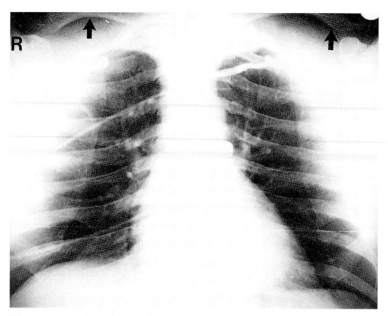

Figure 1.1a   AP radiograph showing the clavicles projected above the lung apices, the scapulae overlying the lung fields, horizontal ribs and magnified heart

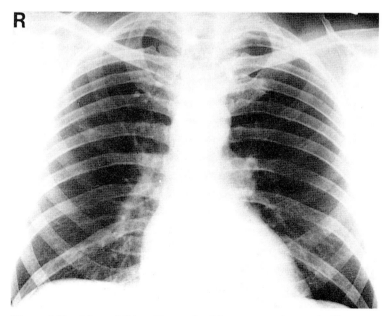

Figure 1.1b   Normal PA radiograph of the same patient as in *Figure 1.1a*

Table 1.1   Essential differences between PA and AP chest radiographs

	PA	*AP*
Heart	Close to film, so little magnification	Magnified image*
Scapulae	Normally rotated away from lungs	Superimposed on lungs
Clavicles	Cross lungs about 5 cm below apices	Frequently projected above lung apices

*The outline of the mediastinum may be widened and distorted. This appearance may mimic aortic aneurysm, for example.

Table 1.2   Normal chest radiograph: features and variations (Fig. 1.2)

● Diaphragm	Smooth outline, convex upwards Right dome is 2 cm higher than the left Usually lies at the level of the 6th rib anteriorly There may be a fat 'pad' adjacent to the cardiac border in obese people A diaphragmatic 'hump' is a normal variant (Fig. 1.3)
● Heart	Transverse diameter of the heart should not exceed half the transverse diameter of the thorax at the level of the diaphragm in the PA projection Geometrical enlargement occurs in the AP radiograph (Fig. 1.1) and apparent enlargement in radiographs obtained in expiration
● Lungs	Degree of transradiancy should be the same on both sides Rotation may produce asymmetry of transradiancy Absence of soft tissues (e.g. breast) will produce increased transradiancy on that side
● Fissures	The horizonal fissure is visible in some adults at the level of the 4th rib anteriorly and merging with the centre of the right hilum Accessory fissures are sometimes visible – azygos, inferior, and rarely a horizontal fissure on the left (Fig. 1.4)
● Lung hila	The left hilum lies approximately 1 cm higher than the right

combination with chest wall abnormalities (e.g. rib fractures).

Increased opacification

Radiologically the normal lung shows branching structures – the pulmonary vessels. These are clearly seen because of the contrast between the relatively opaque blood vessels and the surrounding air-filled lung, which is transradiant. Air-containing bronchi are not normally seen beyond the main bronchi. However, if the alveoli become filled with fluid, either an exudate or a transudate, the lung becomes opaque. In such cases the bronchi, if they remain patent, may be seen as linear transradiancies surrounded by opaque lung – an appearance known as 'air bronchogram'. Tumours or inflammatory masses within the lung also produce opaque areas. If consolidation is present in parts of the lung adjacent to 'solid' structures (e.g. right middle lobe and right heart border), the outline of the solid structure becomes indistinct – the 'silhouette sign' (Fig. 1.7, see p. 28). Some of the causes of lung opacities and their radiological features are summarised in Tables 1.4–1.8.

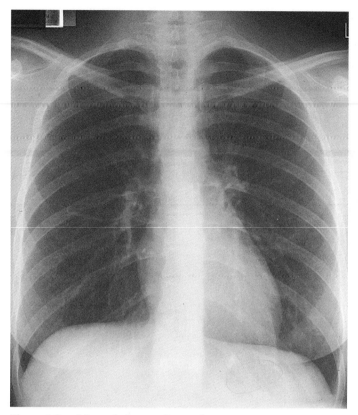

Figure 1.2a   Normal chest radiograph

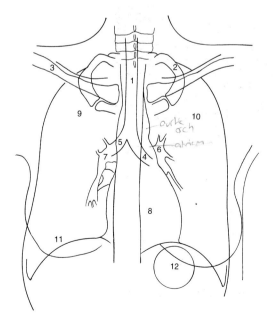

Figure 1.2b   Diagram of the structures shown on a normal chest radiograph:

1. Trachea
2. First rib (left)
3. Right clavicle
4. Left main bronchus
5. Right main bronchus
6. Left hilum
7. Right hilum
8. Heart
9. Right lung
10. Left lung
11. Right hemidiaphragm
12. Air in gastric fundus

(a)

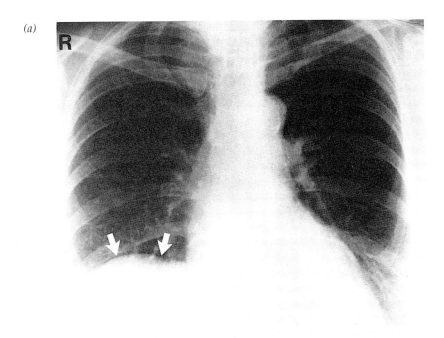

(b)

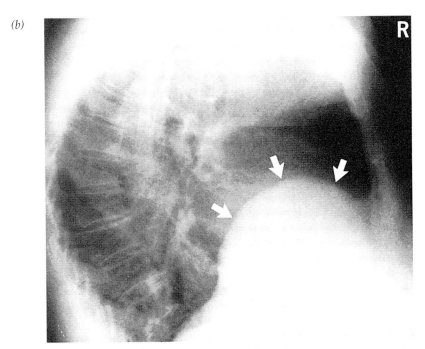

Figure 1.3a and b Anterior 'hump' of the right hemidiaphragm. This has no clinical significance

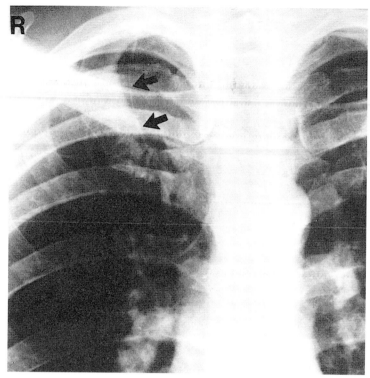

Figure 1.4   Azygos fissure (arrowed)

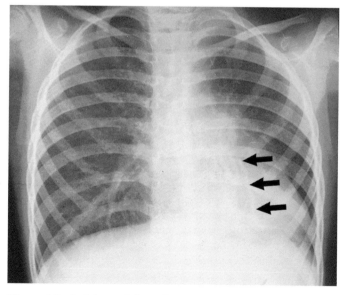

Figure 1.5   Left lower lobe collapse in a child, secondary to bronchiectasis

Table 1.3   Additional chest projections

Projection	Indication
Lateral	To localise opacities or masses
Anteroposterior (erect or supine)	Ill and immobile patients
Penetrated PA	Suspected left lower lobe collapse (Fig.1.5)
Film in expiration	Suspected bronchial occlusion (Fig. 1.6) or small pneumothorax
Lateral decubitus	Possible subpulmonary effusion

(a) *(b)*

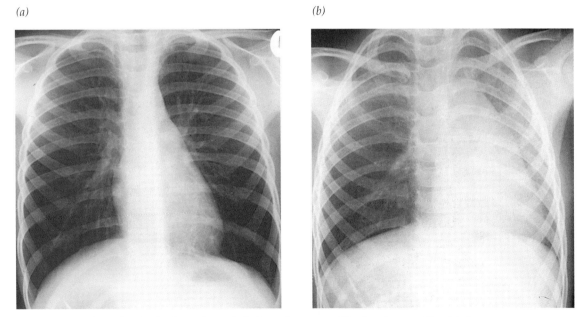

Figure 1.6   Films of a child taken after inhalation of a peanut. The inspiratory film *(a)* shows no abnormality. The expiratory film *(b)* shows evidence of air-trapping on the right, displacing the mediastinum to the left. The peanut was found in the right main bronchus

Table 1.4   Unilateral opacification in the lung

Causes	Radiological features
● Lung collapse secondary to bronchial obstruction (Fig. 1.8) e.g. inhaled foreign body benign neoplasm carcinoma mucus plug	Displacement of the mediastinum towards the side of the lesion. Opacification of affected lobe(s). Elevation of the ipsilateral hemidiaphragm. Displacement of the hilum or fissures towards the area of collapse
● Pleural effusion (Figs 1.9 and 1.10) e.g. congestive cardiac failure malignancy infection following trauma pulmonary infarction hypoproteinaemia	There may be associated features to indicate the cause of the effusion, such as cardiac enlargement, lung mass or nodules, consolidation, etc. A large effusion without mediastinal displacement indicates loss of volume in the contralateral lung. This suggests a carcinoma in adults

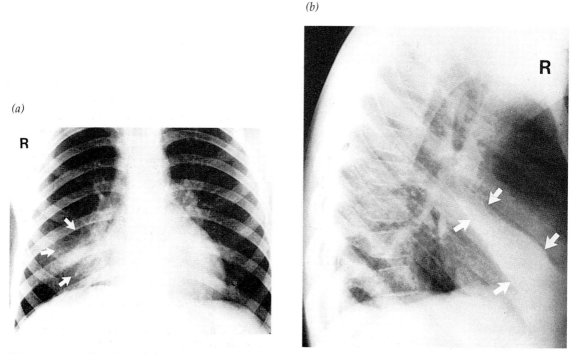

(a)

(b)

Figure 1.7a and b   Consolidation with some collapse of the right middle lobe. Note that the right heart border is obliterated in *(a)* – the 'silhouette sign'

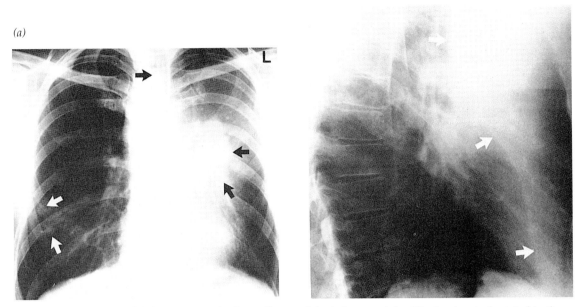

(a)

(b)

Figure 1.8a and b   Left hilar mass producing collapse of the left upper lobe. The trachea is deviated to the left and the oblique fissure on the lateral projection is displaced anteriorly. The left border of the heart is indistinct due to the collapsed lingula. There are metastases in the right lung

Table 1.5   Large opacites in the lungs

Causes	Radiological features
● Pulmonary oedema (Fig. 1.11) e.g. left ventricular failure (due to ischaemic heart disease, hypertension or valve disease) overtransfusion, rapid re-expansion of lung (following aspiration of an effusion)	Left ventricular enlargement usually produces a characteristic outline with displacement of the cardiac apex downwards and laterally. Pulmonary oedema produces diffuse opacification usually extending from the hilar regions which may be indistinct. The upper lobe pulmonary vessels become dilated (venous hypertension). Septal lines and pleural effusions are other features
● Lobar or bronchopneumonia	Opacities of varying size. May be poorly defined or limited to lobar segments. Air bronchogram is sometimes an associated feature
● Pumonary infarction (Fig. 1.12)	Peripheral lung opacities, linear or wedge-shaped, often with small effusion
● Metastases (Fig. 1.13)	Generally rounded opacities varying in size
● Fibrosis e.g. progressive massive fibrosis (PMF) in pneumoconiosis	Associated with multiple small nodules usually. Large opacities may coalesce or cavitate (Fig. 1.14)

(a)

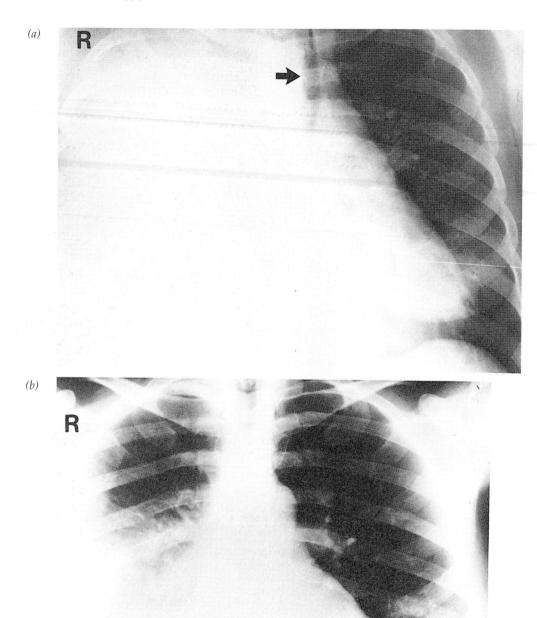

(b)

Figure 1.9a and b   Dense opacity in the right hemithorax due to a large tuberculous pleural effusion in a young female patient. The displaced mediastinal (arrowed) structures return to their normal position as the effusion clears with treatment

(a) *(b)*

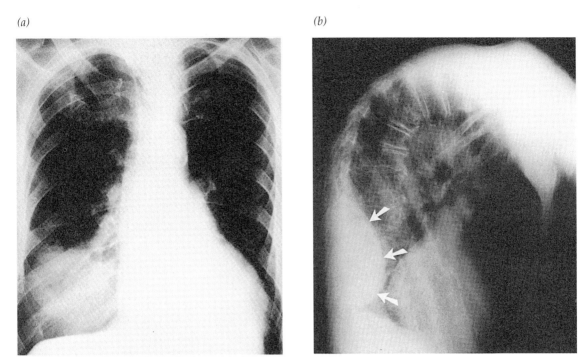

Figure 1.10a and b   Dense, poorly-defined opacity projected in the right lower zone; the lateral projection shows encysted fluid lying posteriorly

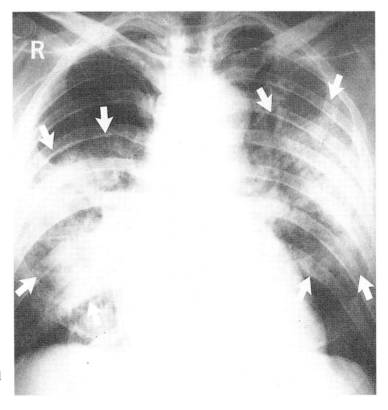

Figure 1.11   Pulmonary oedema. Poorly-defined large areas of opacification. Thickened horizontal fissure due to pleural fluid

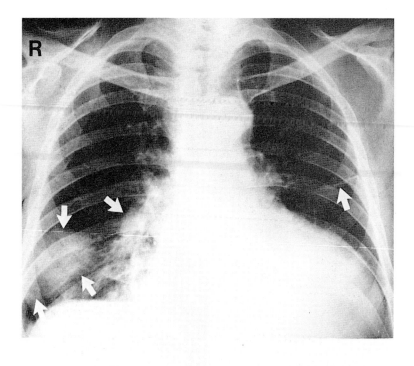

Figure 1.12   Pulmonary infarction. Wedge-shaped opacity at the right base associated with an enlarged pulmonary artery. A linear opacity in the left lung indicates subsegmental collapse and is a common sequel of infarction

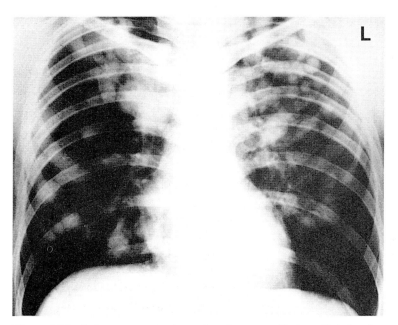

Figure 1.13   Pulmonary metastases showing as multiple well defined, rounded opacities of varying size. The primary site in this case was a teratoma of the testis

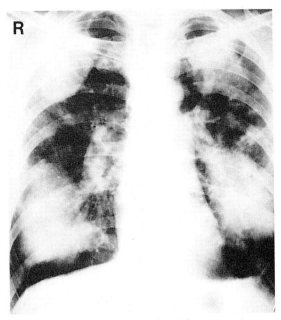

Figure 1.14   Pneumoconiosis with progressive massive fibrosis (PMF). Large, fairly well-defined areas of fibrosis in an ex-miner; background of smaller nodular opacities

Table 1.6   Well-defined rounded opacities in the lungs

Causes	Radiological features

● Single opacities
  e.g. carcinoma or metastases
  (Fig. 1.15)
	Frequently rounded, spiculated (primary tumour) or cavitated

tuberculoma	Frequently calcified with stellate opacities
hamartoma	May show characteristic 'pop-corn' calcification. Rare
mycetoma (Fig. 1.16)	Fungus ball in pre-existing cavity. Thin rim or crescent or air around ball
hydatid cyst	May rupture or become secondarily infected, and a fluid level then appears
pulmonary haematoma	History of trauma. Look for fractured ribs. May cavitate
● Multiple opacities e.g. metastases	Vary in size. Clinical history important
Caplan's syndrome	Combination of pneumoconiosis and rheumatoid arthritis. Background lung nodularity. May cavitate
sarcoidosis (Fig. 1.17)	Hilar adenopathy usually a feature of acute phase. Fibrosis later
hydatid cysts	May be multiple. See above

(a)

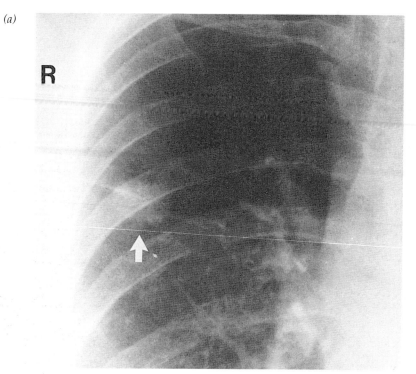

Figure 1.15a   Bronchial carcinoma – small round opacity (arrowed)

(b)

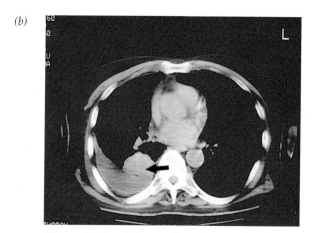

Figure 1.15b   CT scan of a patient with a large bronchial carcinoma in the right lower lobe (arrowed) and an associated pleural effusion

(a)

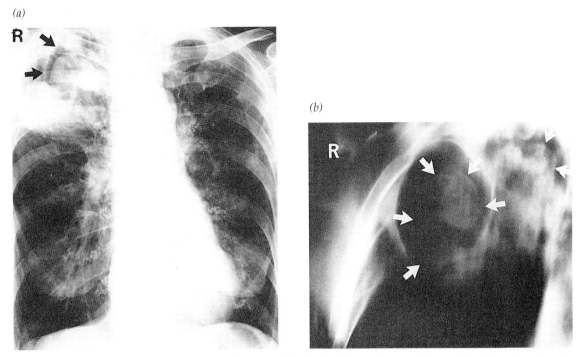

(b)

Figure 1.16a and b   Mycetomas in the right upper lobe. Both hila are elevated due to fibrotic contraction of the upper lobes. Conventional tomography shows the rim of air, or 'halo' sign around the actual fungus ball within each cavity (arrowed)

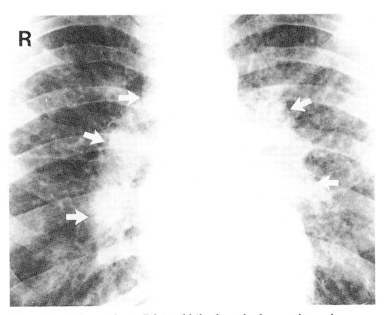

Figure 1.17   Sarcoidosis. Bilateral hilar lymphadenopathy and enlargement of the right paratracheal nodes associated with multiple small nodular pulmonary opacities

Table 1.7   Multiple small opacities up to 5 mm in size in the lungs

Causes	*Radiological features*
● Infections	
Bronchopneumonia	Small ill-defined opacities. Acute history
Miliary tuberculosis	Opacities the size of millet seeds (Fig. 1.18)
● Miscellaneous	
Sarcoidosis	May be associated with hilar/mediastinal lymph node enlargement. Often history of erythema nodosum (Fig. 1.17)
Cystic fibrosis	Microabscesses
Metastases	May resemble miliary tuberculosis or cause 'snowstorm' appearance
● Occupational	
Pneumoconiosis	Small opacities of varying size. Massive fibrosis in upper lobes depending on severity. Hilar nodes may calcify
Extrinsic allergic alveolitis, e.g. Farmer's lung acute stage – dyspnoea and wheeze chronic stage – repeated exposure, increasing dyspnoea	Small nodular opacities throughout lung fields. Severe pulmonary fibrosis leading to cor pulmonale

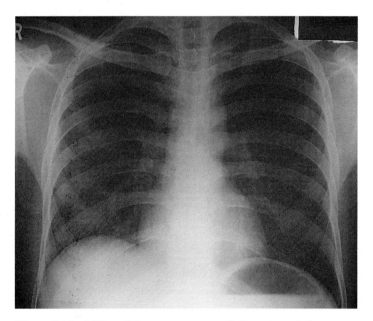

Figure 1.18   Miliary TB – numerous small discrete nodules throughout both lungs, said to resemble millet seeds

Table 1.8   Linear lung opacities*

Causes	Radiological features
● Interstitial pulmonary oedema e.g. left heart failure, valve disease	Short non-branching interstitial or 'septal' lines in the periphery of the lungs (Fig. 1.19)
● Thickened bronchial walls, e.g. chronic bronchitis, cystic fibrosis, asthma, pulmonary oedema	Thin parallel linear shadows seen as rings when projected 'end on'. Are clearly seen on CT (Fig. 1.20)
● 'Fibrous' scars, or areas of persisting sub-segmental collapse, e.g. following previous infection or infarction	Thicker and longer than septal lines; usually basal and directed obliquely across the lung. Common after general anaesthetic and lung or heart surgery
● Lymphatic obstruction, e.g. primary or secondary malignant disease	Associated lung mass. Linear opacities usually radiate from the hila. Associated fine nodularity
● Miscellaneous causes, e.g. pneumoconiosis chronic mitral valve disease	Thickened interstitial spaces, due to fibrosis or deposition of opaque material such as haemosiderosis

*These must be distinguished from normal vascular structures which branch and taper towards the periphery of the lung.

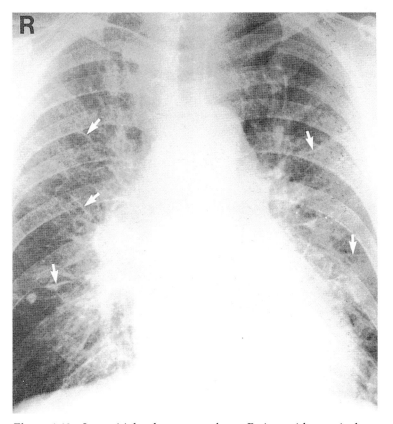

Figure 1.19   Interstitial pulmonary oedema. Patient with ventricular failure and cardiomegaly. The hila are poorly defined

Table 1.9   Localised areas of increased transradiancy in the lungs

Causes	Radiological features
● Cavitation e.g. tuberculosis (Fig. 1.21)	Usually in upper lobes. Cavities due to caseation appear within poorly defined opacities. Calcification later
carcinoma (especially squamous) or metastases (especially sarcoma) (Fig. 1.22)	Cavity usually small in relation to the size of the lesion and often eccentric in position
abscess	Usually follows infection with consolidation. May indicate more proximal bronchial obstruction. May contain fluid level
● Thin-walled bullae	Signs of airways obstruction. Often seen in lung apices
● Pneumatocele e.g. staphylococcal infection	Frequently multiple, thin-walled cavities, may contain fluid. Some persist and predispose to further infections. Risk of associated pneumothorax
cystic fibrosis	Associated with other signs of this disease. Air spaces may be transient and associated with recurrent infections
● Cystic bronchiectasis (Fig. 1.23)	Usually multiple very dilated bronchial 'sacs' in lower lobes. Become secondarily infected

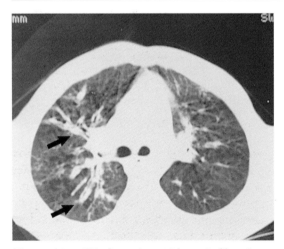

Figure 1.20   CT of a patient with cystic fibrosis, showing dilated thick-walled bronchi (arrowed)

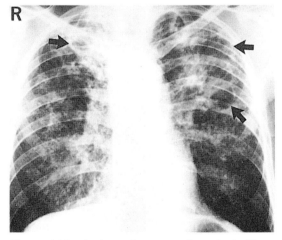

Figure 1.21   Active pulmonary tuberculosis. The disease is mainly in the upper lobes and shows extensive cavitation

Increased transradiancy

Hyperinflation of the lung or parts of the lung or destruction of lung tissue will produce increased transradiancy. This is seen in conditions associated with airways obstruction, such as asthma and emphysema. Abnormal collections of air outside the lung parenchyma, e.g. pneumothorax, will give the same effect. Tables 1.9 and 1.10 outline the radiological features in these situations.

(a)

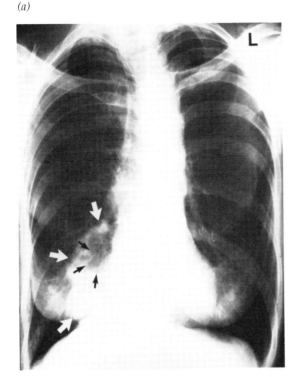

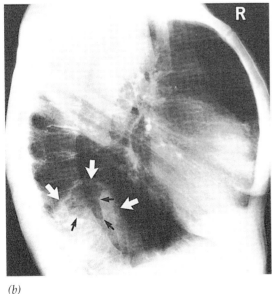

(b)

Figure 1.22a and b Bronchogenic carcinoma. A thick-walled, irregular cavity within the larger mass at the right base

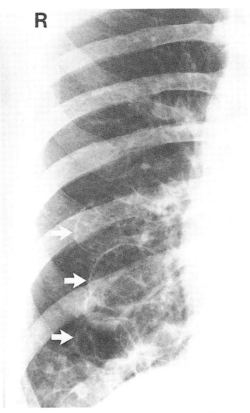

Figure 1.23 Cystic bronchiectasis. Multiple thin-walled 'cysts' in the base of the lung producing a 'soap bubble' appearance. These appear as solid masses if they become infected

The mediastinum

Enlargement of the mediastinal outline may be due to a variety of causes, for instance radiographs obtained with the patient lying supine. Both PA and lateral views may be necessary for localisation of masses. CT is often helpful in giving additional information (Fig. 1.30). The most common causes of a mediastinal 'mass' are aortic dilatation and tortuosity (or aneurysm), hiatus hernia and lymphadenopathy. Other possible causes of mediastinal enlargement should be considered on an anatomical basis, and for this purpose the mediastinum can be conveniently divided into anterior, middle and posterior compartments (Tables 1.11–1.13).

Table 1.10   Large areas of transradiancy in the lungs

Causes	Radiological features
● Obstructive overdistension of a lobe or lung, e.g. inhaled foreign body	Progressively enlarging obstructed lung or lobe causing mediastinal displacement. Requires urgent treatment
● Compensatory overdistension following collapse or removal of part of the lung	Increased transradiancy of remaining healthy lung or lobes
● Airways obstruction e.g. chronic bronchitis or asthma (Fig. 1.24)	Low, flattened diaphragm; narrow vertical heart outline. Lateral film may show anterior bowing of sternum (barrel chest)
● Pneumothorax, either spontaneous or following trauma or surgery, or associated with lung infection and abscess	Air in pleural cavity with variable collapse of underlying lung. Lung 'edge' may be visible (Fig. 1.25). May increase in size to displace mediastinum and cause respiratory distress (tension pneumothorax). May have associated fluid or blood, to give fluid level (Fig. 1.26)
● Vascular causes – diminished pulmonary blood flow or occlusion of pulmonary vessel branches	Pulmonary valve stenosis (in tetralogy of Fallot) leads to oligaemia; thromboembolic disease causes distal 'pruning' of vessels. Diminution in size and number of vessels leads to increased transradiancy
● Chest wall causes, leading to loss of soft tissues	Signs of mastectomy, hemiatrophy (Fig. 1.34)

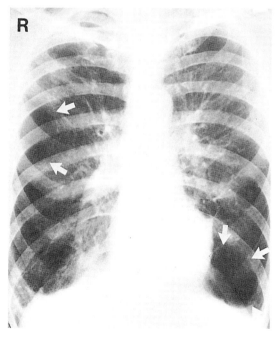

Figure 1.24   Chronic airways obstruction. Narrow vertical heart. Low, flat diaphragm and large pulmonary arteries. Several bullae are present (arrowed)

Pneumomediastinum

This term refers to air in the soft tissue planes of the mediastinum. On a PA radiograph this appears as a linear transradiancy alongside the mediastinal structures, sometimes extending up into the neck, and may also be associated with a pneumothorax or pneumoperitoneum. It occurs occasionally during a severe asthmatic attack and is also an important early sign of perforation of the oesophagus (Fig. 1.31).

The thoracic wall: skeleton and soft tissues

When examining and interpreting a plain chest radiograph it is important to include a careful inspection of the soft tissues and bony structures of the thorax (Fig. 1.32). This will often provide a clue to the nature of disease within the chest (and elsewhere). Injury to the chest may result in fractured ribs, which may in turn lead to a pneumothorax, or haemor-

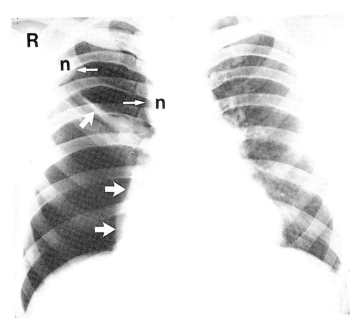

Figure 1.25 Right-sided pneumothorax in a patient with
neurofibromatosis (n). Transradiant hemithorax; the edge of the
collapsed lung is seen adjacent to the right cardiac border, and a
pleural fibrous strand is present in the mid zone

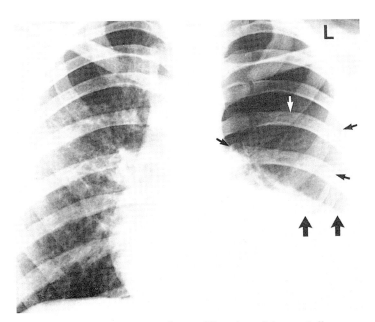

Figure 1.26 Hydropneumothorax. The edge of the partially
collapsed lung may be seen and there are no peripheral lung
markings in the upper part of the left hemithorax

Table 1.11   Abnormalities of the anterior mediastinum

Causes	Radiological features
● Vascular	
Dilated aorta	Very common in older people. It is not usually significant
Aneurysm secondary to:	
atheroma	Frequently seen in elderly subjects. Calcification in aortic knuckle
dissection	Increasing size or aortic outline on serial chest radiographs. May be associated with small left-sided pleural effusion
syphilis	Calcification in the ascending aorta is characteristic (Fig. 1.27)
● Solid masses	
enlarged lymph nodes	Generally have a lobulated outline (Fig. 1.28)
thymoma	Mass in anterior mediastinum may be associated with myasthenia gravis
retrosternal thyroid	Wedge-shaped opacity with apex pointing downwards in the superior mediastinum. Trachea or oesophagus may be displaced and compressed (Fig. 1.29)
● Gastrointestinal	
hernia through foramen of Morgagni (rare)	'Mass' may contain air and/or faeces – i.e. colon. Barium studies will confirm

Table 1.12   Abnormalities of the middle mediastinum

Causes	Radiological features
● Vascular	
Aneurysm of aorta	
Enlarged pulmonary arteries	Project from hila; must differentiate from large lymph nodes. Tomography may be required
● Solid masses	
Enlarged lymph nodes:	Lobulated outline
reticulosis	May be associated with lymphadenopathy elsewhere
sarcoidosis	Usually well defined, bilateral and symmetrical. Lung signs later
secondary carcinoma	

(a)

(b)

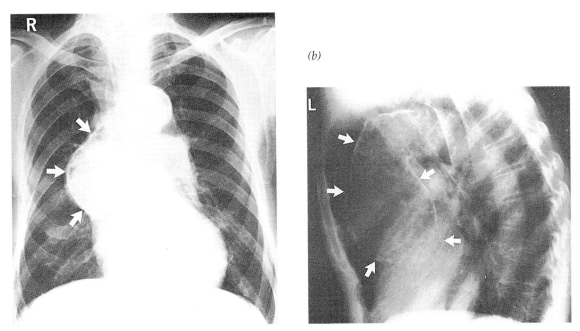

Figure 1.27a and b Aneurysm of the ascending aorta, shown on the PA film as a mass obscuring the right hilum. Calcification in the wall of the aneurysm extending from the aortic valve to the arch

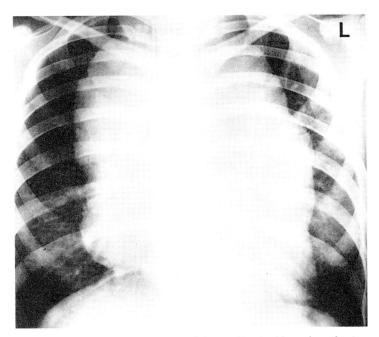

Figure 1.28 Gross enlargement of the mediastinal lymph nodes in a patient with lymphosarcoma

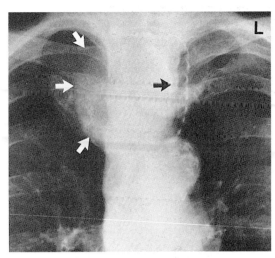

Figure 1.29   Retrosternal thyroid displacing the trachea to the left

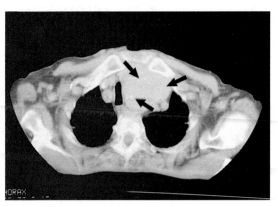

Figure 1.30   CT scan showing a mediastinal mass (arrowed) compressing and deviating the trachea to the right. The mass contains foci of calcification (open arrows). Diagnosis: retrosternal goitre

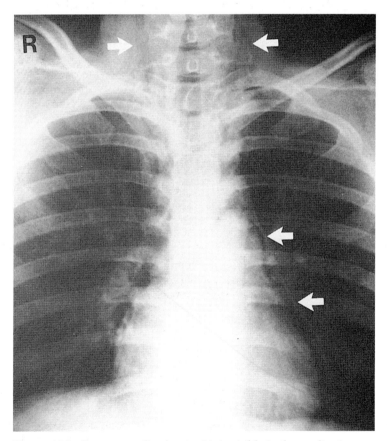

Figure 1.31   Pneumomediastinum. Air is visible in the mediastinum, around the aortic knuckle and can be seen tracking up into the soft tissues of the neck. This patient had spontaneous rupture of the oesophagus

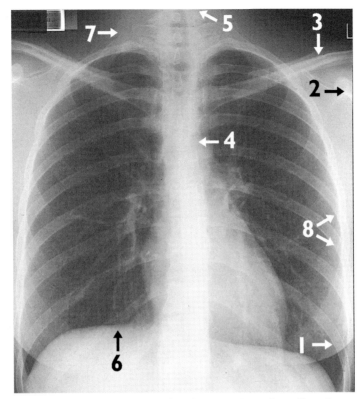

Figure 1.32   Key: 1 Outline of the breast; 2 Scapula; 3 Clavicle; 4 Thoracic spine; 5 Cervical spine; 6 Diaphragm; 7 Soft tissues of the neck; 8 Ribs

Table 1.13   Abnormalities of the posterior mediastinum

Causes	Radiological features
● Gastrointestinal	
Hiatus hernia	Gas-containing structure often superimposed on the heart on the PA radiograph and may contain a fluid level
Achalasia	Enlargement to the right of the mediastinum from diaphragm upwards, sometimes simulates a large heart. An air–fluid level high in the mediastinum may be present
● Spinal	
Infection:–	
e.g. tuberculous, pyogenic	Destruction of vertebral body, narrowing of disc space adjacent. Paravertebral opacity due to abscess; may be multicentric
neurofibromata	Evidence of neurofibromatosis elsewhere. Enlargement of intervertebral foramina – 'dumb-bell' tumour
neurenteric cyst	Well-defined rounded mass. Frequently associated spinal abnormality, which may be in cervical region

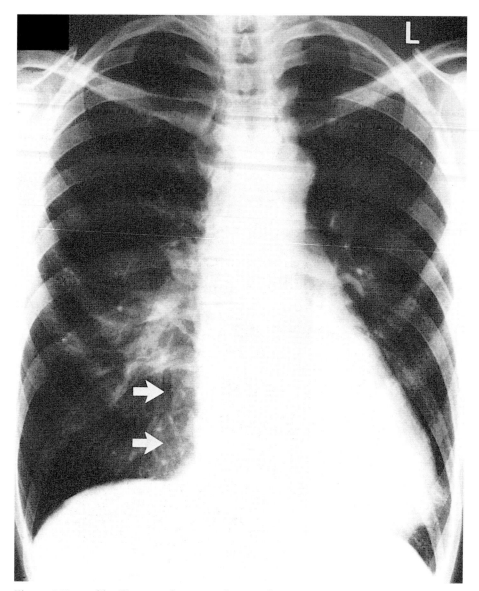

Figure 1.33a and b   Depressed sternum (arrowed)

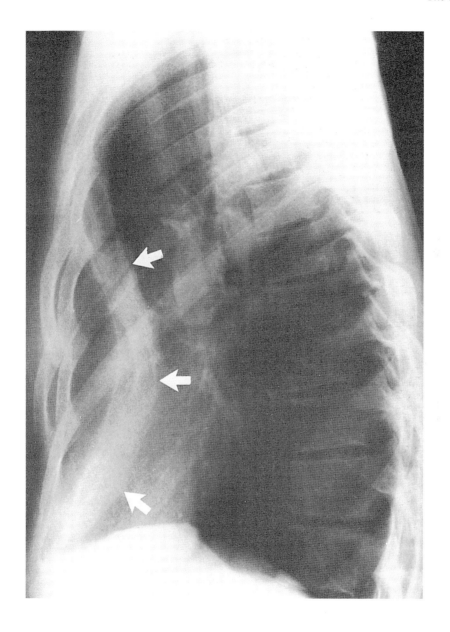

rhage into the thoracic cavity. The latter resembles a pleural effusion radiologically. Minor congenital rib anomalies, such as anterior fusion or bifid ribs, are relatively common and are of no clinical significance. Congenital depression of the sternum, or pectus excavatum, gives typical radiological signs, such as loss of the outline of the right heart border, apparent increased opacification at the right cardiophrenic angle, straightening of the left heart border and steep oblique angulation of the anterior ends of the ribs (Fig. 1.33). Further examples of important chest wall lesions are shown in Figure 1.34. Some of the radiological signs shown here may mimic intrapulmonary disease and lead to incorrect interpretation of the radiograph.

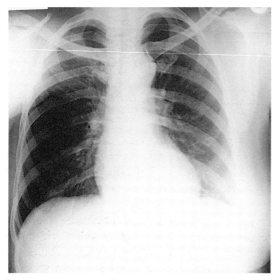

Figure 1.34a Right mastectomy with associated soft tissue swelling (lymphoedema) of the right arm

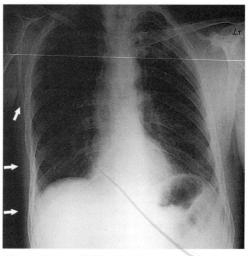

Figure 1.34b Polio. Hemiatrophy affecting the right side of the body

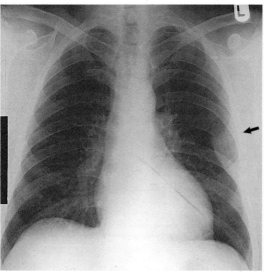

Figure 1.34c Pathological rib fracture (arrowed) in myelomatosis. Note the soft tissue component of the lesion

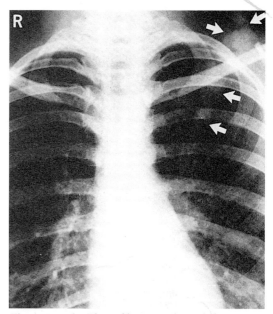

Figure 1.34d Plait of hair overlying left apex. This could be misinterpreted as an abnormality

Chapter 2

The cardiovascular system

The major components of the cardiovascular system shown on a chest radiograph are (1) the heart, (2) the aorta and (3) the pulmonary circulation (Fig. 2.1). Abnormalities of these structures may be broadly classified into:

- enlargement of the cardiac outline
- cardiac chamber enlargement – shunts and valve disease
- enlargement of the great vessels
- changes in the pulmonary vasculature.

The radiological signs of cardiac failure have been described in Chapter 1 (Fig. 1.11).

Radiographs of the abdomen and pelvis may show calcification and enlargement of the abdominal aorta and its branches. Calcified peripheral arteries may be seen in radiographs of the limbs. Otherwise, more specialised techniques are necessary to show abnormalities of the vascular system.

Enlargement of the heart

Cardiac measurement on plain radiographs is imprecise and minor degrees of cardiac or chamber enlargement cannot be assessed. As a rough guide, if the maximum transverse diameter of the heart exceeds half the transverse diameter of the thorax at the level of the diaphragm the heart is assumed to be enlarged. Abnormalities of the cardiac outline other than overall enlargement are sometimes useful and may indicate specific cardiac abnormalities such as valve disorders. Severe ischaemic heart disease usually causes non-specific cardiac enlargement accompanied by signs of cardiac failure. It is possible to identify enlargement of individual cardiac chambers on a chest radiograph under certain circumstances. However, a complex combination of radiological signs may be present because the haemodynamic effects of valve disease and congenital cardiac shunts, for instance, usually affect more than one chamber and may also affect the pulmonary circulation.

An example of a complex radiological picture is chronic mitral valve disease. The overall heart size is often normal but the left atrium is dilated and the left atrial appendage is visible beyond the left heart border (Fig. 2.2). Incompetence of the valve tends to produce considerable enlargement of both left-sided chambers, sometimes with calcification of a giant left atrium. The chest radiograph may eventually show signs of pulmonary venous hypertension, with dilated upper lobe veins and constriction of lower lobe vessels (so-called 'vascular redistribution'), pulmonary oedema (alveolar and interstitial) and, rarely, osseous pulmonary nodules.

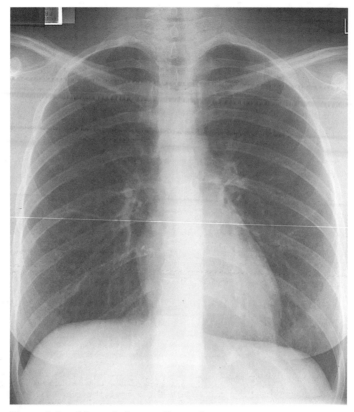

Figure 2.1a   Normal chest radiograph

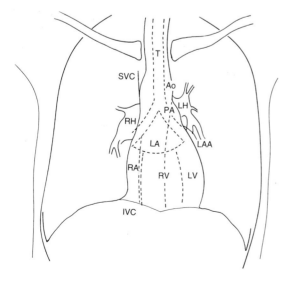

Figure 2.1b   Diagram showing cardiac chambers
and major vascular structures:

Ao	Aortic Knuckle
SVC	Superior Vena Cava
PA	Main trunk of the pulmonary artery
RH	Right hilum
LH	Left hilum
LA	Left atrium
LAA	Position of left atrial appendage
RA	Right atrium
RV	Right ventricle
LV	Left ventricle
IVC	Position of inferior vena cava

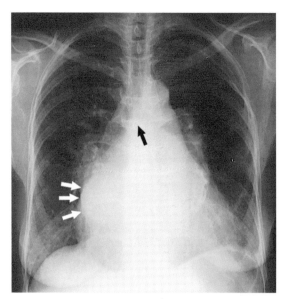

Figure 2.2 Mixed mitral valve disease. Note the enlarged left atrium, splaying the carina and causing an apparent double right heart borner (arrowed)

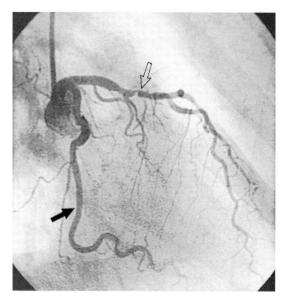

Figure 2.3a Left coronary angiogram. Note the stenosis in the left anterior descending artery (arrowed). The other vessel is the circumflex artery (open arrow)

Echocardiography is useful in the further assessment of cardiac abnormalities such as valve disease, cardiac tumours (rare) and pericardial effusion. The technique provides additional qualitative information about cardiac function and flow. Radionuclide imaging contributes to the assessment of cardiac ischaemia; thallium scans are used to demonstrate areas of reversible ischaemia and multiple gated acquisition (MUGA) scans give an assessment of cardiac function. More recently MRI has played an increasing part in the assessment of cardiac function, particularly in the presence of congenital heart lesions. Coronary angiography and left ventricular contrast studies are the mainstay of the investigation of ischaemic heart disease and are invariably performed before coronary artery bypass graft surgery (Fig. 2.3).

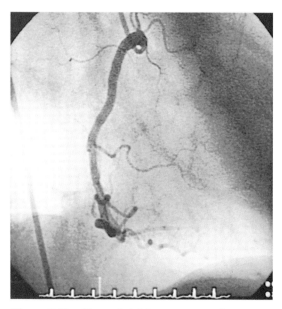

Figure 2.3b Normal right coronary angiogram

Pericardial effusion

A large pericardial effusion will cause enlargement of the cardiac outline (Fig. 2.4); however, the radiographic signs are not specific and cannot usually be differentiated

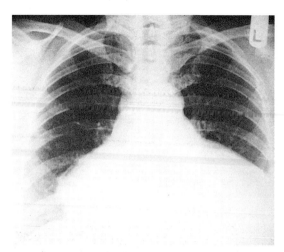

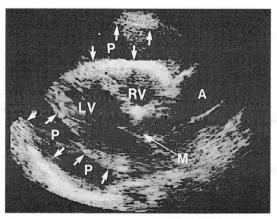

Figure 2.4b   Real time ultrasound scan through the right ventricle (RV)

Figure 2.4a   Large cardiac silhouette due to a pericardial effusion

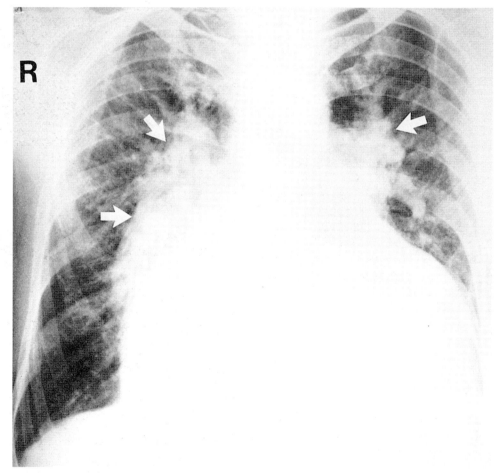

Figure 2.5   Atrial septal defect in an adult – gross cardiomegaly, markedly enlarged proximal pulmonary arteries with constriction peripherally indicating reversal of shunt (Eisenmenger's syndrome)

from those of cardiac enlargement due to other causes. A rapid change in the size and shape of the cardiac outline between consecutive chest radiographs is one useful indicator, provided that the radiographs are technically satisfactory and comparable. Sonographic confirmation is then necessary (Fig. 2.4). Pericardial calcification may occur as a late complication of acute pericarditis and effusion, and is best seen on a lateral radiograph of the chest.

The pulmonary circulation

Increase in the size of the pulmonary vessels occurs in a variety of conditions, especially left-to-right cardiac shunts such as atrial and ventricular septal defects (Fig. 2.5). It is sometimes difficult to distinguish between enlarged pulmonary arteries and veins when the more central vessels are involved, but the arteries form the more superior elements of the lung hila, and the veins the lower elements (entering the left atrium below the level of the carina). High cardiac output states such as thyrotoxicosis or pregnancy may cause a generalised but reversible increase in the size of the pulmonary vessels.

In pulmonary venous hypertension (usually due to left-sided cardiac failure) there is specific and characteristic dilatation of the upper lobe veins. Pulmonary arterial hypertension due to thromboembolic occlusive disease affecting the distal pulmonary vessels results in marked dilatation of the central pulmonary arteries with 'pruning' of more distal vessels. The same feature is also seen in the Eisenmenger syndrome (Fig. 2.5).

The aorta

Plain radiographs of the chest and abdomen may give some indication of aortic enlargement; signs include mediastinal widening, mural calcification, and central or paracentral abdominal mass (usually fusiform). Further investigations are necessary to give more accurate information. Ultrasonography is useful in confirming the presence of an abdominal aneurysm and in the follow-up of already diagnosed aneurysms to monitor signs of enlargement. CT or MRI are usually used to demonstrate the full extent of an aneurysm and to detect complications such as dissection and rupture (Fig. 2.6).

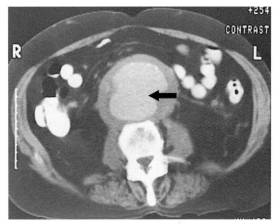

Figure 2.6a   CT scan of an abdominal aortic aneurysm (arrowed)

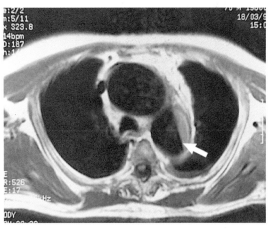

Figure 2.6b   Axial MRI scan of a dissection of the thoracic aorta. The dissection flap is arrowed

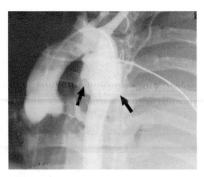

Figure 2.6c Angiogram showing traumatic transection of the aorta (arrowed)

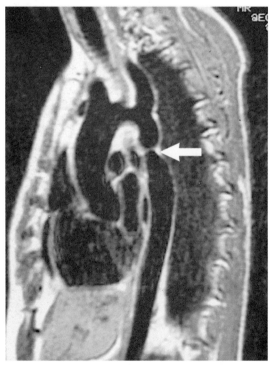

Figure 2.6d Sagittal oblique MRI scan of congenital coarctation of the aorta (arrowed)

Peripheral vascular disease

Peripheral blood vessels are not visible on plain radiographs unless their walls are calcified. Initial non-invasive assessment of the peripheral arterial system is now performed using duplex ultrasound techniques, which

show the presence of atheromatous plaques causing stenoses and occlusions and also give information about abnormalities of flow caused by such lesions.

Arteriography must be performed to localise and to assess the extent of vascular disease more accurately. The femoral artery is usually used for access; it is punctured under local anaesthetic and a catheter is introduced into the vessel over a guide wire under fluoroscopic control. Water-soluble contrast medium is then injected under pressure and a rapid sequence of radiographs of the region under review is obtained. A conventional arteriogram is shown in Figure 2.7. This tech-

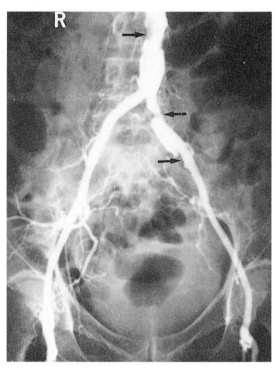

Figure 2.7 Angiogram showing extensive atheroma involving lower aorta and iliac vessels. Plaques and stenoses are present; both internal iliac arteries are occluded

nique has been largely replaced by digital subtraction angiography (DSA). Here the images are processed to delete unnecessary background anatomical detail, such as bony structures, in order to enhance the clarity and

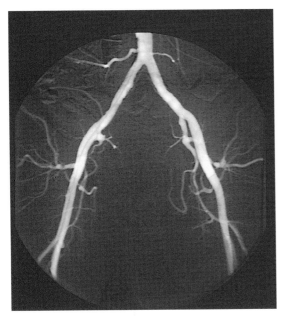

Figure 2.8   Digital subtraction angiogram of the aortic bifurcation and iliac vessels

(a)

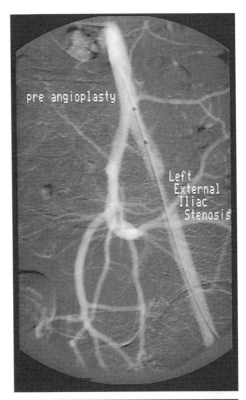

(b)

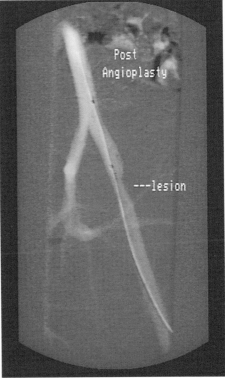

detail of the blood vessels being examined (Fig. 2.8).

During percutaneous revascularisation techniques a wire is placed across the stenosis or occlusion in the artery, followed by a small catheter. When angioplasty is being used the catheter contains a deflated balloon which is positioned across the stenosis; the balloon is then inflated to dilate the vessel, restoring its lumen (Fig. 2.9). In some cases an expanding metallic stent is left in position to maintain the patency of the vessel (Fig. 2.10).

A history of sudden onset of pain in a limb, followed by pallor, decreased skin temperature and absent peripheral pulses, clinically indicates an embolic episode. Arteriography will localise the site of the embolus and thrombolytic agents may then be infused directly into the obstructed vessel to restore patency (Fig. 2.11).

Figure 2.9   Left external iliac stenoses: (*a*) before and (*b*) after angiooplasty

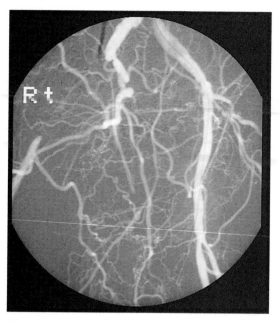

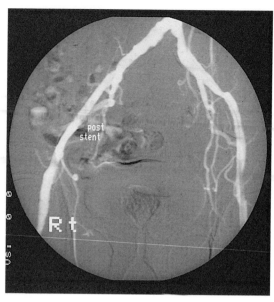

Figure 2.10a   Angiogram showing occlusion of the right external iliac artery

Figure 2.10b   Following insertion of a metal stent; patency of the vessel is restored

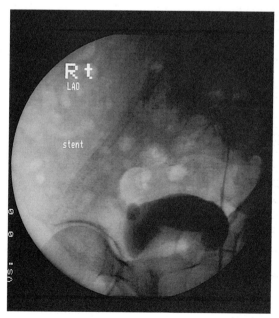

Figure 2.10c   Unsubtracted view to show the stent

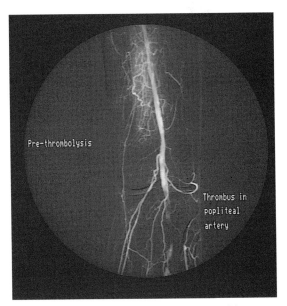

Figure 2.11a   Patient presenting with sudden onset of cold, painful, white lower leg. The popliteal artery is occluded

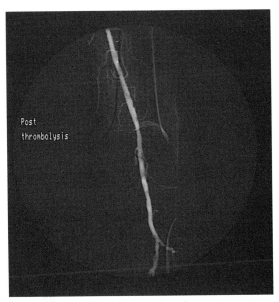

Figure 2.11b   Following infusion of tissue plasminogen activator (TPA) the thrombus cleared and the artery became patent

The venous system

The most common reason for examining the veins is in the investigation of possible deep vein thrombosis in the lower limbs. Duplex ultrasonography is the preferred investigation for demonstrating this abnormality and should be used whenever the appropriate equipment and operative expertise is available. Contrast venography is performed when the results of duplex scans are equivocal (Fig. 2.12). Other parts of the venous system can also be examined in this way, e.g. the inferior vena cava, the upper limb veins and the superior vena cava. Compression and obstruction of the superior vena cava is the usual indication for an upper limb venogram (Fig. 2.13). Studies of the inferior vena cava are indicated when thrombosis or compression by an abdominal mass is suspected.

Repeated episodes of pulmonary infarction by emboli originating in the lower limb or pelvic veins cause serious management problems, especially when adequate coagulation therapy has apparently been maintained. Caval filters can be placed in the inferior vena cava under fluoroscopic and venographic control to prevent further pulmonary emboli. These devices are radio-opaque and expand within the inferior vena cava, giving an umbrella-like appearance (Fig. 2.14).

The lymphatic system

In the past, lymph vessels and nodes were outlined by injecting an oil-based iodine-containing contrast medium into lymph vessels in the dorsum of the foot. Placing the needle and infusing up to 10 ml of contrast medium sometimes took several hours to perform. The contrast medium remained in regional lymph nodes for several months and allowed follow-up of abnormal nodes using plain radiographs. This technique has been replaced almost completely by radionuclide lymphangiography. Here, a radioactive small-particle colloid is injected into the foot and images of the lymphatic system are obtained

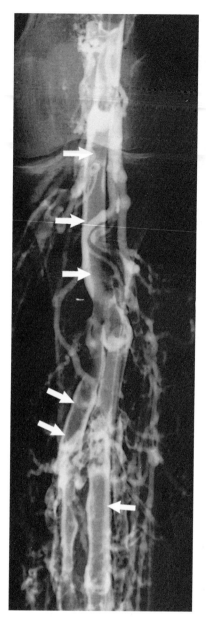

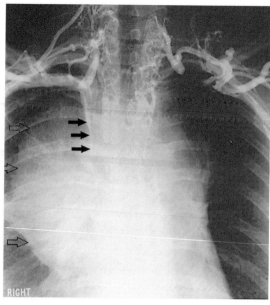

Figure 2.13 Bilateral upper limb venography showing almost complete occlusion of the superior vena cava (arrowed) due to a large mediastinal mass (open arrows)

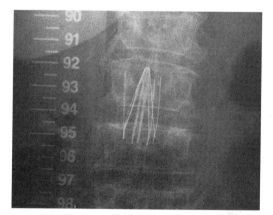

Figure 2.12 Contrast venogram of the lower limb showing extensive thrombus within the deep veins of the calf and the popliteal vein

Figure 2.14 Inferior vena cava filter. The ruler was used to help position the filter accurately

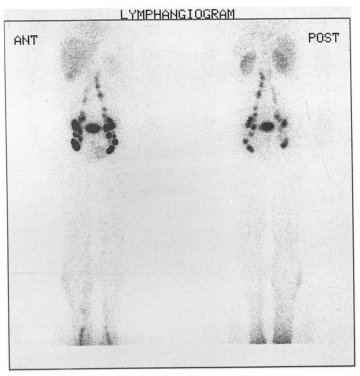

Figure 2.15 Normal isotope lymphangiogram. This image was obtained 3 hours after injection of the isotope and shows the pelvic lymph nodes

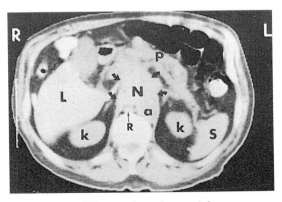

Figure 2.16 CT scan – lymphoma. A large mass of nodes (N) surrounds the aorta (a) and displaces vessels and the pancreas (p) anteriorly. An enlarged retrocrural node (R) is also seen. 'L' represents liver, 'S' spleen and 'k' kidneys

some time later (Fig. 2.15). The technique is useful in cases of suspected lymphatic obstruction. Contrast lymphography and radionuclide scanning have been used in other parts of the body to study regional lymphatic drainage.

CT and MRI provide excellent non-invasive means of assessing lymph node enlargement (Fig. 2.16). This now forms part of the assessment and staging of malignant tumours of all kinds and provides a more comprehensive picture of the spread of malignant disease, particularly as there are significant 'blind' areas in conventional lymphography, e.g. the internal iliac nodes are not outlined in lower limb studies.

Chapter 3

The abdomen and alimentary tract

The normal plain abdominal radiograph

The plain radiograph of the abdomen may present difficulties in interpretation because the contents of the abdominal cavity have similar soft tissue densities and, unlike the structures of the chest, are not sharply outlined by air, with the exception of some parts of the gastrointestinal tract. Use is made instead of the fat layer that surrounds some of the abdominal organs. Fat is less dense than soft tissues and appears as transradiant stripes around organs such as the kidneys. The gas that normally lies within the gastro-intestinal tract may give useful information about the presence of disease. Some normal structures in the abdomen calcify; in other situations the calcification is pathological. Calcification is clearly visible on plain radio-graphs because of its relatively high density.

Other structures included on the abdominal radiograph, such as lung bases and parts of the skeleton, should also be carefully studied. These structures often given important infor-mation about the possible cause of a patient's symptoms and may provide coincidental, but possibly significant, information about other non-abdominal areas and systems.

A supine abdominal radiograph obtained in the radiology department under optimal conditions gives more useful information than any other projection. Additional views, including the erect, give only complementary information and are indicated only in special circumstances. These alternative projections should therefore not be requested in isolation. Portable radiographs of the abdomen rarely give useful information and should be avoided.

A chest radiograph should always be obtained in patients presenting with suspected acute abdominal disorders. Some chest conditions, e.g. pneumonia, may present with referred abdominal pain, especially in childhood.

The following account of abdominal abnor-malities will focus on two main radiological features: gas patterns and abdominal calcifica-tion.

Gas patterns

Normal abdominal radiographs

In the supine abdominal radiograph gas is normally present in the body of the stomach and in variable amounts in the transverse and other parts of the colon. It is also present in small amounts in the small intestine of adults. Normal gas–fluid levels are usually seen in the gastric fundus on erect radiographs and occasionally in the first part of the duodenum and in the caecum. In infants and children gaseous distension of the stomach and of the intestines is a common feature. In infants in particular this is largely due to swallowed air. Supine abdominal radiographs occasionally show apparent soft tissue masses in the gastric fundus or duodenal loop; these are well-recognised 'pseudo-tumours' and are due to normal fluid collections gravitating to these dependent areas.

Abnormal gas patterns

Abnormal gas patterns in abdominal radiographs may be conveniently classified into:

- excessive intestinal gas
- abnormal contour of gas-containing loops
- extraluminal gas.

Tables 3.1–3.3 summarise the important features.

Abdominal calcification

Many structures in the abdomen calcify, especially in older subjects; most of these are of no clinical significance. They include the walls of blood vessels, lymph nodes and costal cartilages. Calcification may also occur in pathological states but may be discovered coincidentally. Gallstones and prostatic calcification fall into this category. Those that are often associated with symptoms include calcified urinary calculi, pancreatic calcification (Fig. 3.7) in chronic pancreatitis, and calcification occurring in abdominal tumours.

Radiological examination of the gastrointestinal tract

Contrast studies of the gastrointestinal tract and endoscopic diagnostic techniques play complementary roles in the investigation of

Table 3.1   Excessive intestinal gas

Causes	Radiological features
● Physiological Air swallowing, usually in children	Non-specific gaseous distension. No consistent end-point to suggest obstruction
● Mechanical obstruction Small bowel, e.g. adhesions, hernia, Crohn's disease	Gaseous distension of loops of small bowel which lie centrally. Valvulae conniventes visible. Short fluid levels on erect film (Fig. 3.1)
Large bowel, e.g. carcinoma, diverticular disease with stricture	Distension of peripherally situated large bowel, proximal to obstruction. Haustra visible. Longer fluid levels than in small bowel (Fig. 3.2)
Volvulus of the caecum, sigmoid	Specific radiological signs. Extremely dilated loops extending upwards from normal site of these structures to lie in upper quadrants. Very long fluid levels in erect film
● Non-mechanical obstruction (or 'pseudo-obstruction') Generalised ileus, e.g. following surgery, peritonitis, metabolic disorders	Large and small bowel distended. May resemble mechanical obstruction
Localised ileus e.g. appendicitis, pancreatitis, abscess, ischaemia	Single loop of dilated bowel (sentinel loop). Speckled gas in abscess

(a)

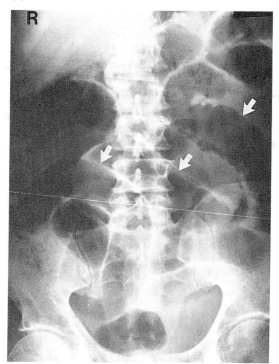

(b)

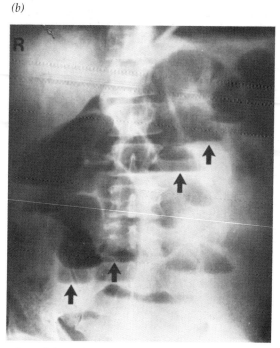

Figure 3.1 *(a)* Small bowel obstruction. Distended loops of small bowel. Valvulae conniventes are present in the jejunum (left upper quadrant) but the ileum is featureless in comparison. *(b)* The erect film shows numerous air/fluid levels

Table 3.2 Abnormal contour of gas-containing loops

Causes	Radiological features
● Crohn's disease	Affects small or large bowel, or both. Stricture may be visible, or irregularity of mucosa due to ulceration. May show signs of obstruction or toxic megacolon (see below)
● Ulcerative colitis	Narrowed, featureless empty colon. Pseudopolypi may be visible as filling defects. Gross dilatation – 'toxic megacolon' – is a dangerous complication (Fig. 3.3) and predisposes to perforation
● Ischaemia	Dilated bowel, thickened wall with areas of oedema – 'thumb-printing' (Fig. 3.4). Ileus, with signs of obstruction (Table 3.1)
● Intrinsic masses	Tumours and intussusception may be outlined by gas
● Displaced loops	Large non-alimentary abdominal masses, e.g. enlarged spleen, may displace or indent gas-filled loops of otherwise normal bowel

(a)

(b)

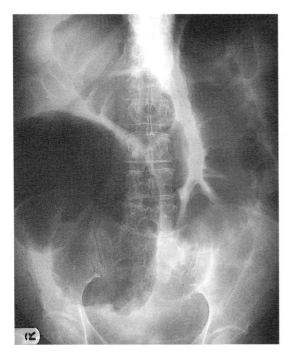
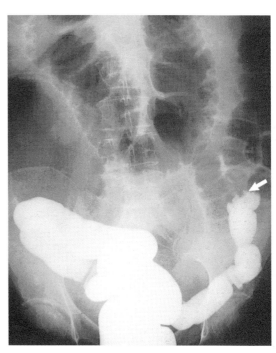

Figure 3.2 *(a)* Dilated gas-filled loops of large bowel indicating obstruction of the large bowel. *(b)* Limited single-contrast barium enema in the same patient, showing the site of obstruction in the distal descending colon (arrowed)

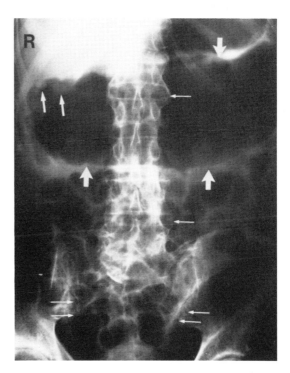

Figure 3.3 Toxic megacolon. Patient with ulcerative colitis. Markedly dilated transverse colon, loss of the normal haustral pattern. Pseudopolyps are shown in the region of the hepatic flexure. Note also associated changes of sacro-iliitis and ankylosis of the spine

Table 3.3   Extraluminal gas

Causes	Radiological features
● Intraperitoneal	
Perforation of a hollow viscus	Variable amounts of gas, from small crescent under diaphragm (erect film) to gross peritoneal distension
Subphrenic abscess	Air–fluid level under diaphragm. Adjacent lung base consolidation. Confirm with ultrasound (Fig. 3.5)
● Bowel wall	
Infarction, necrotising enterocolitis in infants	Linear streaks of gas in bowel wall. May coalesce or outline portal vein radicles (Fig. 7.9)
Pneumatosis coli	Blebs of gas in colon wall. Symptoms may mimic carcinoma. Usually elderly patient with airways obstruction
● Biliary tree	
After sphincterotomy or anastomosis between biliary tree and bowel	Branching gas pattern in liver (bile ducts). Usually lie centrally in liver; gas in portal vein radicles extends more peripherally
Erosion of gallstone into small bowel; erosion of duodenal ulcer into biliary tree; pancreatic neoplasm; gas-forming infection	Small bowel obstruction ('gallstone ileus') and opaque calculus may be visible in intestine with gas in biliary tree (Fig. 3.6). Other causes listed do not cause intestinal obstruction
● Genitourinary tract	
Fistula, e.g. trauma, postoperative, Crohn's disease	Gas may outline urinary bladder, ureters and collecting systems. Differential diagnosis: gas-forming infection in diabetic patients

alimentary tract symptoms. How these different methods are deployed in different hospitals depends to a large extent on the availability and accessibility of endoscopy. Hospitals with comprehensive endoscopy facilities and 'open access' policies tend to use this technique as the first-line investigation in patients with gastrointestinal symptoms. This has been accompanied by a decline in the numbers of barium studies carried out in the same hospitals. In general, patients complaining of dysphagia can be investigated using either endoscopy or radiology: dyspepsia is investigated by endoscopy; colonic symptoms are investigated using barium techniques, followed by colonoscopy for further clarification and biopsy; upper gastrointestinal bleeding (haematemesis and melaena) is investigated with endoscopy; the small bowel is examined by means of a specialised barium technique. There will be many local variations in the way that some of these investigations are used.

Barium examinations

Barium sulphate suspensions are specially formulated for use in different parts of the alimentary tract. Whether they are taken orally or introduced through small bowel or rectal tubes, they are accompanied by gas (carbon dioxide) releasing agents or air insufflation to produce what is known as air contrast or double contrast. This allows detec-

(a)

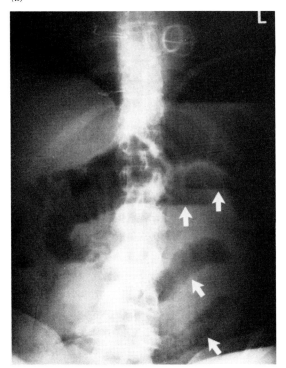

(b)

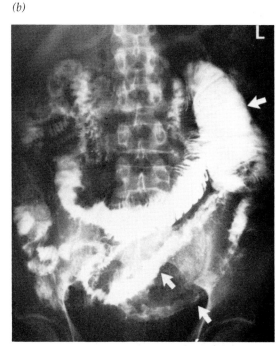

Figure 3.4 *(a)* Ischaemia of small bowel. Patient with a prosthetic mitral valve who developed occlusion of the superior mesenteric artery due to an embolism. The erect plain abdominal radiograph shows fluid levels in small bowel with abnormal contour of gas containing loops in the left lower quadrant. *(b)* Barium examination shows the markedly dilated jejunum and evidence of mucosal oedema with 'thumb-printing' in the more distal narrowed small bowel

tion of small mucosal lesions as well as improving the accuracy of these techniques in detecting masses, polyps, strictures, infiltrations and surface erosions and ulceration.

All barium examinations are carried out under fluoroscopic control to optimise mucosal barium coating and gaseous distension. Assessment of gut distensibility and motility can also be made during fluoroscopy. Biopsy techniques have been used in conjunction with barium studies of the oesophagus but have not gained widespread acceptance. Endoscopic ultrasound techniques are becoming established and have been shown to be useful in the oesophagus, stomach and rectum. Contrast examination of the small bowel will be discussed in a later section in this chapter.

In this section it is appropriate to discuss radiology of the alimentary tract according to the clinical presentation – dysphagia, dyspepsia, bleeding, symptoms suggesting small bowel disease, and large bowel disorders.

Dysphagia

This is a common symptom. Its radiological assessment often requires a rapid sequence of radiographs or video recording during fluoroscopy, so that the swallowing function can be studied in detail from the oropharynx to the gastric cardia. The common causes of dysphagia and their radiological features are summarised in Table 3.4.

Dyspepsia

This term is used to describe upper abdominal

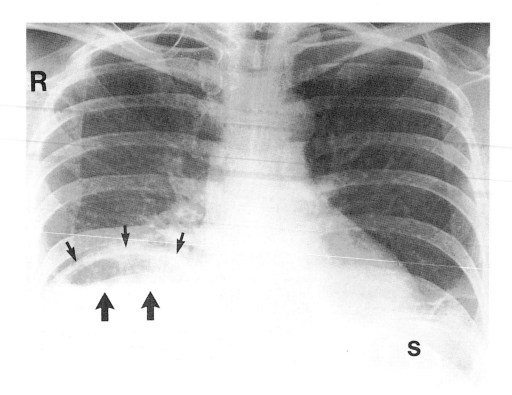

Figure 3.5   Subphrenic abscess. Air-fluid level under the elevated right hemidiaphragm with consolidation at both lung bases

symptoms arising from a variety of different conditions. Epigastric pain, with or without a relationship to food, is an extremely common symptom. Peptic ulceration, hiatus hernia with gastro-oesophageal reflux, gastric neoplasm and diseases of the biliary tract (e.g. gallstones) and pancreas (e.g. chronic pancreatitis, carcinoma) all tend to cause similar symptoms. It is possible to distinguish between these conditions to some extent on the basis of symptom complexes, particularly their relationship to meals. Persistence of symptoms despite adequate medical treatment, weight loss, vomiting, blood loss (haematemesis and melaena), persistent pain with radiation away from the typical site of peptic ulcer or gallstone pain are all features that give cause for concern. In this situation the patient should be investigated intensively,

using endoscopy as the first investigation. If endoscopy is negative, radiological techniques, including plain abdominal radiographs, upper gastrointestinal barium studies and ultrasonography, are used, depending on the symptom complex. Ultrasonography is useful for the detection of biliary and pancreatic disease; CT may be added to complete the investigations by outlining areas not demonstrated by ultrasonography, e.g. the retroperitoneal planes.

Uncomplicated dyspepsia which is short lived is usually managed conservatively (particularly in young adults) using one of the many anti-dyspepsia drug regimens. The decision to investigate this common problem depends on the availability of endoscopy services. There is, however, some debate about the appropriateness of the current

Table 3.4   Dysphagia

Causes	Radiological features
● Post-cricoid carcinoma	Irregular narrowing; mass displacing larynx forwards (Fig. 3.8)
● Pharyngeal diverticulum	Variable size, arising posteriorly
● Oesophageal web	Characteristic appearance; associated with iron-deficiency anaemia (Fig. 3.9)
● Malignant stricture	May be primary oesophageal cancer or invasion by bronchial or mediastinal tumour. Characteristic appearance – irregular narrowing, 'shouldering', partial or complete obstruction
● Stricture secondary to reflux oesphagitis and hiatus hernia complex	Reflux shown during fluoroscopy; mucosal ulceration, hiatus hernia; strictures tend to be smooth but may mimic carcinoma (Fig. 3.10)
● Achalasia	Generalised motility defect with dysfunction of cardia causing obstruction and sometimes gross dilatation of oesophagus, with food and liquid residue
● Miscellaneous causes: corrosive strictures	Severe ulceration initially. Tendency to perforate
moniliasis, herpes infection	Opportunistic infection. Severe ulceration and pain
systemic sclerosis	Impaired peristalsis
neurological disorders	Swallowing difficulties with aspiration into lungs

widespread use of endoscopy in this particular clinical circumstance.

Barium meal

The standard double-contrast study of the upper gastrointestinal tract includes views of the oesophagus, stomach and duodenum. The examination is carried out following a period of starvation; peristalsis is temporarily abolished using an injection of glucagon or an atropine-like agent. This enhances mucosal coating with barium suspension and allows detection of small mucosal lesions, e.g. erosions and polyps. The radiographs obtained are examined for evidence of ulceration, deformity, infiltration, stricture formation, external compression or displacement,

and obstruction. Some of the radiological abnormalities that may be found are summarised in Table 3.5.

The major advantage of endoscopy in the investigation of alimentary disorders is the ability of the operator to obtain biopsies of lesions or suspicious mucosal abnormalities. Sources of bleeding can also be identified accurately. Endoscopy is not without complications and it has been claimed that good barium studies are as accurate as endoscopy in the detection of significant lesions.

What has become apparent over recent years is that many benign and malignant diseases of the gastrointestinal tract cause similar or identical radiological signs, and that some benign lesions become, or harbour, malignant disease. Disorders such as achala-

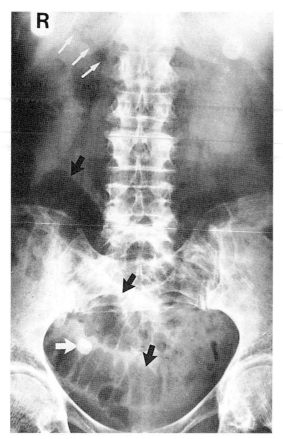

Figure 3.6 Gallstone ileus. Note laminated gallstone in the right iliac fossa and dilated small bowel loops – gas is present in the biliary tree. The opacity in the left upper quadrant is a button in the patient's clothing

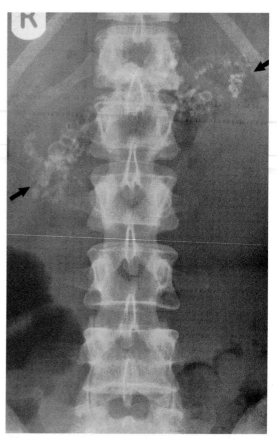

Figure 3.7 Pancreatic calcification (arrowed) indicating chronic pancreatitis

sia, peptic and corrosive strictures of the oesophagus, gastric ulcers and certain non-epithelial sub-mucosal tumours, such as leiomyomas, predispose to, or undergo, malignant transformation into malignant tumours. Therefore direct inspection of the lesions, obtaining biopsies where necessary, is an accepted way of following up some lesions such as gastric ulcers. It is also known that malignant ulcers undergo cyclical healing changes and may therefore mimic benign ulcers.

Finally, benign ulcers may cause marked localised fibrosis and deformity when they heal. This change is usually permanent and should not be the sole justification for further follow-up using barium studies.

Gastrointestinal bleeding

Bleeding may be the first manifestation and presenting feature of gastrointestinal disease. The clinical picture may vary from severe haematemesis to anaemia due to occult blood loss (e.g. cancer of the stomach or colon), melaena or frank rectal bleeding. Careful questioning may pin-point other symptoms, and clinical examination may reveal signs that help to localise the cause of the bleeding. Very occasionally no cause is found after exhaustive investigation and these patients may require exploratory operations.

Endoscopic techniques are the preferred method of investigation because the sources of bleeding, both in the upper gastrointestinal tract and in the colon, can be identified.

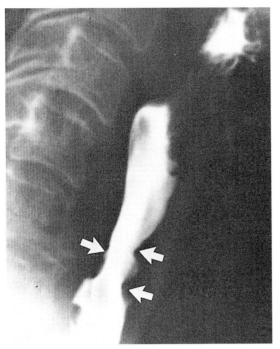

Figure 3.8 Post cricoid carcinoma – an irregular filling defect encircling the upper oesophagus

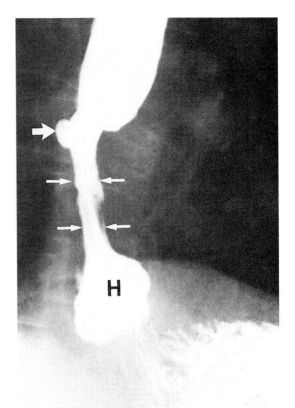

Figure 3.10 Benign peptic stricture of the lower oesophagus in a patient with a hiatus hernia (H). Note also the presence of an ulcer crater (larger arrow)

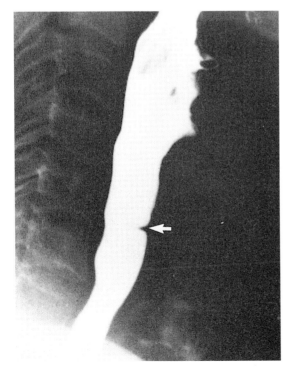

Figure 3.9 Oesophageal web – appears as a constant sharp indentation on the anterior aspect of the upper oesophagus

Table 3.5   Dyspepsia

Causes	Radiological features
● Oesophageal disease: hiatus hernia complex	Superficial mucosal ulceration in the oesophagus indicates oesophagitis. Reflux may be detected but barium studies are less sensitive than endoscopy or pH studies. Strictures may develop and may be indistinguishable from malignant strictures (Fig. 3.10)
● Gastric abnormalities: ulceration (Figs 3.11, 3.12)	Barium collection in crater. Radiating folds of mucosa to edge of crater. Surrounding deformity and oedema. Heal to form distinctive scars. May be malignant from outset. Careful endoscopic follow-up necessary, with biopsies
polyp(s)	Multiple polyps in body of stomach form part of chronic gastritis spectrum – usually hyperplastic in nature, and benign. Adenomatous polyps, usually in antrum, may be premalignant lesion(s). Should be removed. Other types of polyps may be part of familial polyposis syndromes
cancer (Fig. 3.13)	Characteristic signs in advanced disease. Either ulcerating or polypoid, or mixture of both. Early or superficial cancers resemble benign ulcers but with specific signs such as 'clubbed' mucosal folds and geographical areas of very superficial ulceration
non-mucosal tumours	Usually large and may have surface ulceration or excavation. Exogastric extension. May be leiomyoma, sarcoma or lymphoma
● Duodenal disease: e.g. ulceration (Fig. 3.14)	Characteristic ulcer crater(s) in first part of duodenum, with deformity. Atypical signs in Crohn's disease and Zollinger–Ellison syndrome

Barium studies may show the causal abnormality but may also show unrelated diseases, which may cause confusion. Barium persisting in the alimentary tract may preclude the use of more effective investigations, such as isotope-labelled red blood cell scans or selective coeliac and mesenteric angiography (Fig. 3.17), to localise sites of bleeding beyond the reach of diagnostic endoscopy, or when the latter is 'negative'. Table 3.6 lists some causes of upper gastrointestinal bleeding and their radiological features. It is important to remember that bleeding may arise in the small bowel or in the caecum; these areas are not easily accessible during endoscopy. Furthermore, bleeding may be intermittent, and may vary in severity from sub-clinical to catastrophic and life threatening. All diagnostic methods are more accurate during active bleeding. Angiography must be carried out when bleeding is brisk (a rate of over 5 ml/min is often quoted); isotope-labelled red blood cell scans may detect slower rates of bleeding but are anatomically less precise (Fig. 3.17).

Selective coeliac and mesenteric angiography is time consuming and is rendered more difficult and hazardous if the patient's general condition is deteriorating due to the rate of blood loss. The technique may show a vascular lesion or demonstrate extravasation of contrast medium into the bowel lumen.

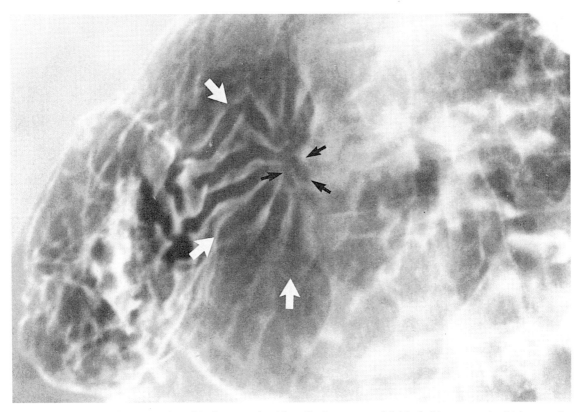

Figure 3.11   Healed gastric ulcer (black arrows) with rediating mucosal folds (white arrows) which extend up to the ulcer crater, suggesting that the lesion is benign. Endoscopic follow-up would nevertheless be considered

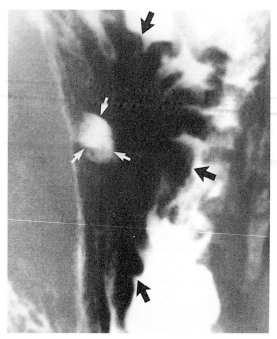

Figure 3.12   Gastric ulcer crater surrounded by abnormal, thickened mucosa and rugal folds. This is a malignant ulcer confirmed by endoscopy

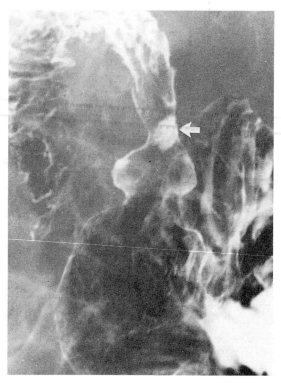

Figure 3.14   Duodenal ulceration associated with deformity of the first part of the duodenum (the 'cap' or 'bulb').

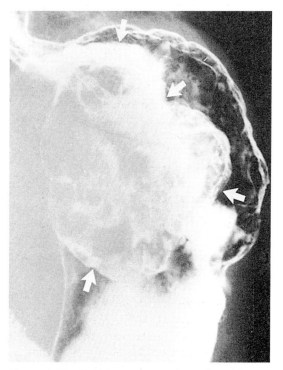

Figure 3.13   Gastric carcinoma. Large irregular polypoid filling defect in the fundus and body of the stomach

Table 3.6   Upper gastrointestinal bleeding

Cause	Radiological features
● Oesophagus	
Varices due to portal hypertension	Serpiginous filling defects on barium studies of the lower oesophagus (Fig. 3.15)
Mucosal tear following vomiting (Mallory–Weiss lesion)	Tears rarely shown radiologically. Endoscopy preferred
Oesophagitis, all causes	Endoscopy more sensitive. Barium studies may show ulceration
● Stomach	
Erosions	Characteristic multiple 'target' lesions (Fig. 3.16). Acute or chronic gastritis
Ulcer, tumour, varices	Characteristic appearances (Table 3.5). Varices here usually accompanied by varices in the oesophagus, though not invariably
● Duodenum	
Ulceration, invasion from adjacent tumour	Characteristic findings in duodenal ulceration; signs of malignant infiltration also characteristic

In a patient with portal hypertension it may be important to demonstrate the patency of the portal vein if shunt procedures are being considered. Delayed radiographs will demonstrate the venous phase of an angiogram and will outline draining and collateral veins. This technique has superseded the hazardous direct approach of splenoportography which involved direct needle puncture of the spleen.

One cause of rectal bleeding, particularly in childhood, is a Meckel's diverticulum. Because this contains gastric mucosa which ulcerates and bleeds, it is readily detectable using a technetium isotope scan. The ectopic gastric mucosa is shown as a localised area of increased isotope activity, usually lying centrally in the abdomen.

The small intestine

The usual indications for investigating the small intestine are:

● abdominal pain, weight loss, diarrhoea – symptoms suggesting inflammatory disease;
● colicky abdominal pain, distension, vomiting – symptoms suggesting obstruction, which may be intermittent;
● anaemia, malabsorption – caused by a variety of small bowel disorders.

Abdominal radiographs may show signs of small bowel obstruction but the cause may not be apparent. Evidence of inflammatory disease in the colon is helpful (Table 3.2).

Small bowel contrast studies may be a continuation of a barium meal (a 'follow-through' study) although the high density barium contrast agent used specifically for double-contrast studies of the oesophagus, stomach and duodenum may give poor images of the small bowel. For the small bowel a large volume of relatively low density

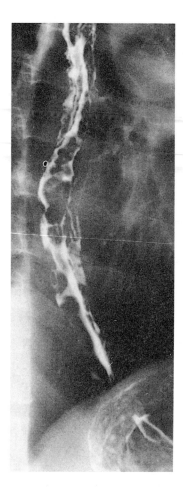

Figure 3.15   Irregular filling defects in the oesophagus due to large oesophageal varices in a patient with portal hypertension

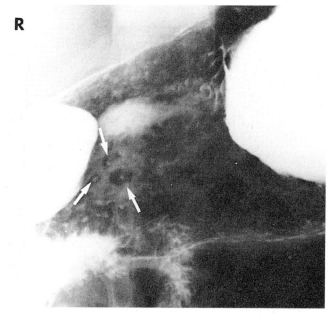

Figure 3.16   Gastric erosions in the antrum appearing as small flecks of barium surrounded by transradiant 'halos'

Table 3.7 Small bowel disorders

Causes	*Radiological features*
● Crohn's disease	Signs of bowel inflammation – characteristic fissuring or 'rose-thorn' ulcers, nodular or 'cobble-stone' mucosa, strictures, thickened bowel wall, adherence of adjacent loops, fistulae to adjoining structures, 'skip' lesions, dilated and obstructed loops of bowel, involvement of stomach, duodenum and colon. Terminal ileum is commonly affected, but disease may be extensive (Fig. 3.18)
● Obstruction due to causes other than inflammation	Small bowel contrast studies usually localise site of obstruction provided proximal loops are not too distended. Adhesions produce characteristic deformities of affected loops, especially when using small bowel enema technique
● Malabsorption problems, other than those caused by inflammatory disease	Coeliac syndrome causes non-specific dilatation of small bowel loops in severe cases but small bowel biopsy is much more specific. Jejunal diverticulosis (Fig. 3.19), blind loops, fistulae and strictures may all cause malabsorption and are detectable on contrast studies

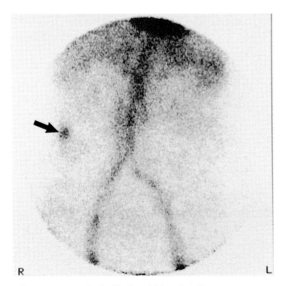

Figure 3.17a Labelled red blood cell scan showing accumulation of isotope at the site of a bleed in the ascending colon (arrowed)

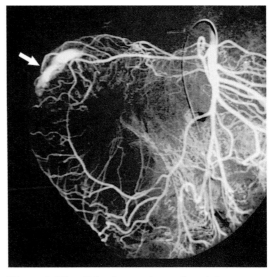

Figure 3.17b Selective angiography of the superior mesenteric artery demonstrating a bleeding point in the middle colic artery territory (arrowed)

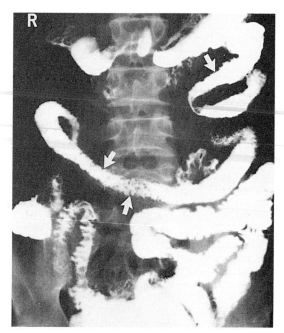

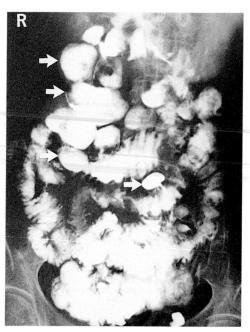

Figure 3.18   Extensive small bowel involvement due to Crohn's disease shown on a barium follow through examination. The abnormalities include deep ulceration and 'cobblestoning' of the mucosa

Figure 3.19   Multiple small bowel diverticula

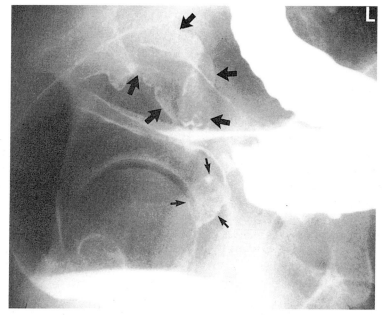

Figure 3.20   Large irregular malignant polyp shown on the posterior rectal wall in a patient presenting with rectal bleeding. The smaller polyp seen anteriorly was benign histologically (small arrows)

Table 3.8 Common disorders of the large intestine

Causes	*Radiological features*
● Carcinoma	Most are irregular strictures with 'shouldering'. Destroyed mucosal pattern, proximal dilatation and obstruction. Invasion of adjoining tissues and organs. May appear as polyp, usually more than 2 cm with complex surface pattern (Fig. 3.20). Long-standing ulcerative colitis and familial polyposis coli are predisposing conditions
● Diverticular disease	Multiple diverticula particularly in sigmoid region, but may be widespread. Narrowing and deformity. Common, so may coexist with cancer. May bleed or perforate, or form fistulae, e.g. with bladder
● Ulcerative colitis	Diffuse, uniform fine ulceration; loss of haustra, giving featureless tubular colon (Fig. 3.21). Toxic megacolon (Fig. 3.3) and carcinoma are complications. May only involve distal colon or rectum in some cases
● Crohn's disease	Areas of narrowing, deep ulceration, strictures. Perianal disease is common. Prone to form fistulae. Coexists with small bowel disease often
● Ischaemic colitis	Cause of profuse bleeding and acute abdominal pain. Narrowing of lumen, often affecting localised segment, with mucosal oedema ('thumb-printing'). Occasionally difficult to distinguish from Crohn's disease

(semi-transparent) barium suspension is more appropriate.

A more detailed study of the small bowel may be indicated if a follow-through examination is inconclusive; this consists of administering the barium suspension via a catheter introduced through the mouth into the proximal small intestine (small bowel enema, or enteroclysis). This method has some well-documented advantages but is more invasive. Fluoroscopy is used to determine the optimal infusion rate of contrast agent and allows 'spot films' of areas of interest to be obtained during the infusion.

The radiological features of some common small bowel disorders are summarised in Table 3.7.

The large intestine

Symptoms such as altered bowel habit, rectal bleeding, abdominal pain, weight loss and anaemia may indicate serious colonic disease. Colonoscopy and barium studies are complementary and equally useful but their deployment depends to a large extent on the availability of colonoscopy services. Many clinicians use the barium enema as the first-line diagnostic investigation and either combine this with flexible fibreoptic sigmoidoscopy or reserve a full colonoscopy for those instances where a barium study is inconclusive or where a lesion shown radiologically requires further direct examination and biopsy.

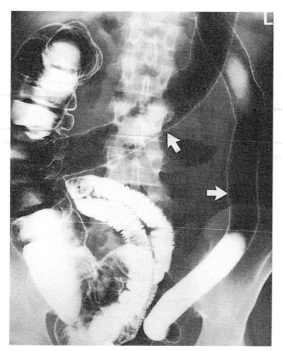

Figure 3.21a Barium enema examination – appearances typical of ulcerative colitis. Fine mucosal ulceration and loss of normal haustral pattern shown in the descending and transverse colon

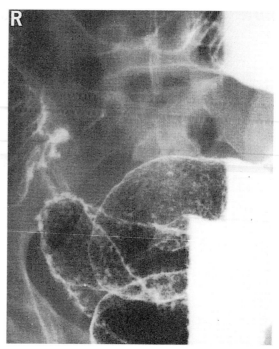

Figure 3.21b Extensive ulceration involving the rectum and lower sigmoid colon in a patient with ulcerative colitis

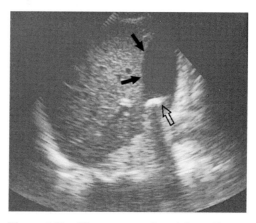

Figure 3.22 Ultrasonography of the gall bladder (black arrows) containing a gallstone (open arrow). The structure shown adjacent to the gallbladder is the liver

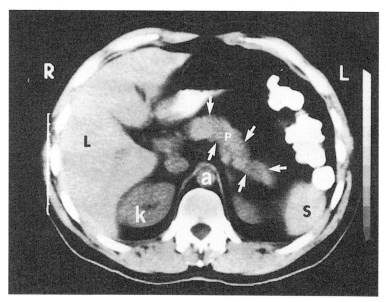

Figure 3.23 CT scan through the upper abdomen demonstrating a normal pancreas, 'P'. The liver 'L', spleen 'S', right kidney 'k' and aorta 'a', are also shown

Barium studies require full bowel preparation using one of a variety of cleansing techniques (faecal residue may mimic polyps or tumours). A double-contrast technique involves inflation of the colon using air or carbon dioxide, and peristaltic activity is temporarily abolished using a short-acting atropine-like pharmacological agent.

Colonoscopy provides direct access to lesions or suspicious areas of mucosa for biopsy; small polypoid lesions may be amenable to removal during the same diagnostic procedure. The examination may not be complete because in a significant proportion (10–30%) the caecum is not reached and there are also 'blind' spots at points of angulation of the colon. Advanced diverticular disease produces deformity and narrowing that is difficult to assess both in barium studies and during colonoscopy.

Colonoscopy has a significantly higher risk of complications than barium enema, and the procedure is more time consuming.

Table 3.8 summarises the radiological features of common disorders of the large intestine.

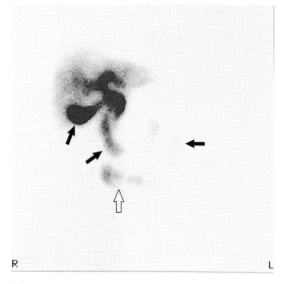

Figure 3.24 Normal HIDA scan. At 35 minutes after the injection the tracer has passed through the liver and biliary tree into the small bowel (arrows). The gallbladder is also shown (open arrow)

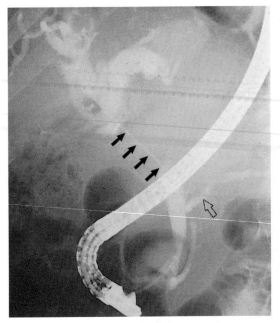

Figure 3.25a   ERCP demonstrating a stricture of the common hepatic duct with dilatation of the intra-hepatic ducts. A cannula has been passed across the stricture (arrows). The pancreatic duct (open arrow) is not shown in its entirety but is normal

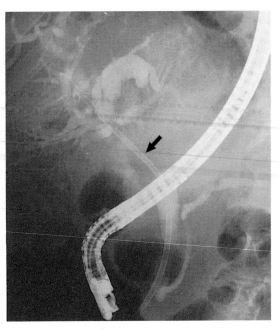

Figure 3.25b   A stent has been placed across the stricture to allow bile drainage

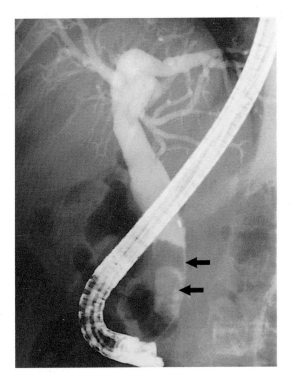

Figure 3.25c   ERCP showing calculi in the common bile duct (arrowed). Baskets and balloon catheters are used to remove such calculi following enlargement of the Sphincter of Oddi by diathermy

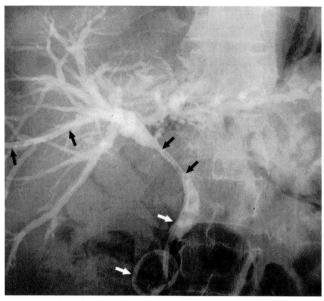

Figure 3.26 A drain (black arrows) has been placed percutaneously across a biliary stricture (position marked with open arrows) and into the duodenum. Side-holes in the drain above and below the stricture allow bile to pass into the duodenum

Liver, biliary tract and pancreas

Ultrasonography is the first-line investigation and has almost completely replaced oral cholecystography for the demonstration of gallstones (Fig. 3.22). Signs of acute cholecystitis can be detected: mural thickening, oedema and surrounding fluid. Ultrasonography also demonstrates the bile ducts (which become dilated if the lower, distal end is obstructed by a calculus, primary tumour or pancreatic tumour), the liver parenchyma (e.g. metastatic deposits) and the head of the pancreas, provided that there is no intervening intestinal gas.

CT and MRI are used to investigate the liver and the pancreas (Fig. 3.23), giving greater detail of any lesion(s) and indicating extension into adjacent tissues or organs.

Radionuclide imaging is useful in two specific circumstances. Acute cholecystitis may be demonstrated by technetium-using compounds of iminodiacetic acid, such as labelled HIDA; occlusion of the cystic duct prevents the isotope from collecting in the gall bladder and the latter is shown as a 'cold' area, devoid of radioactivity, on the scan. HIDA scans are also used to demonstrate abnormalities of biliary drainage (e.g. obstruction of extrahepatic ducts, where no isotope reaches the bowel), and bile leaks, usually following surgery or trauma (Fig. 3.24).

When abnormalities of the pancreatic or bile ducts are suspected, endoscopic retrograde cholangiopancreatography (ERCP) (Fig. 3.25) is used to demonstrate strictures (benign or malignant) or impacted bile duct calculi. This technique also allows access to the ducts for stone removal or for insertion of obstruction-relieving stents (Fig. 3.25). This latter procedure is used as a palliative measure in inoperable bile duct or pancreatic neoplasms.

An alternative approach to the management of bile strictures, benign or malignant, is percutaneous insertion of a drain or stent, as shown in Figure 3.26.

Chapter 4

The genitourinary system

Radiological examination of the genitourinary tract

Some information about the genitourinary system may be obtained from plain abdominal radiographs, e.g. enlargement or shrinkage of the kidneys, distension of the bladder, opaque calculi in the urinary tract, calcification other than calculi – nephrocalcinosis, bladder wall calcification. Gas in the urinary tract has a very distinctive appearance; calcification in parts of the genital tract also produces characteristic signs – uterine fibroids and prostatic and seminal vesicle calcification can be identified easily.

The genitourinary system is investigated using ultrasonography in the first instance. The technique gives information about the site, size and shape of the kidneys, the condition of the collecting systems and renal parenchyma, and also the female genital tract. A distended bladder forms a good acoustic window for the examination of pelvic structures.

A detailed sonographic examination of the urinary bladder is important and the findings may determine if a patient needs further direct examination of the bladder by fibre-optic or rigid cystoscopy.

Excretion urography (intravenous pyelography, IVP; intravenous urography, IVU) involves an intravenous injection of water-soluble iodinated contrast agent (see Part 1). As there is a finite risk of an adverse reaction to these agents this investigation should not be undertaken without valid clinical justification. Since ultrasonography has taken over the primary role in the radiological investigation of the genitourinary tract, excretion urography is generally reserved for the demonstration of the collecting systems and ureters. Following the intravenous injection of contrast medium, abdominal radiographs are obtained at approximately 5 minute intervals for up to 20 minutes in order to outline sequentially the upper tracts, the ureters and the bladder (Fig. 4.1). Localised radiographs of the renal areas and alternative projections of other parts of the urinary tract can be interposed, depending on the initial findings. Enhanced detail of the renal anatomy is obtained by using conventional tomography. Obstruction causes delay in the excretion of contrast medium (Fig. 4.1) and therefore the examination may be extended over a longer period of time (so-called 'delayed films'). Excretory urography gives more information about the site of obstruction than ultrasonography. A control radiograph of the abdomen is necessary before excretory studies are carried out because opaque contrast medium may obscure calcified calculi.

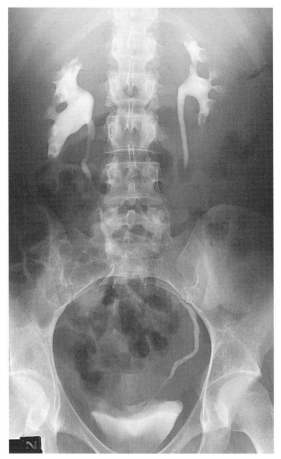

Figure 4.1a Normal excretory urogram – non-obstructed pelvicalyceal systems and ureters 15 minutes after the injection of contrast medium

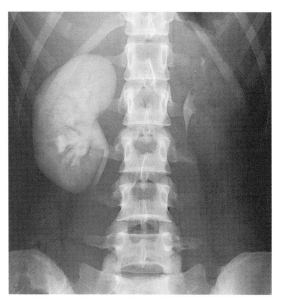

Figure 4.1b Patient with right-sided renal colic. Note the delayed nephrogram on the right side, with obstruction of the ureter at about the level of the fourth lumbar vertebra due to a calculus. The left kidney is normal

CT of the genitourinary tract is carried out as part of a tumour staging process – for renal, retroperitoneal, bladder and other pelvic neoplasms in particular. It is often helpful to include a contrast phase to outline the collecting systems, ureters and bladder and this is therefore an adaptation of excretory urography.

More specialised contrast studies of the genitourinary tract may be carried out under certain circumstances.

Antegrade pyelography

This procedure is performed by puncturing the renal collecting system percutaneously and is used in patients with hydronephrosis (detected by ultrasonography or excretory urography) due to distal obstruction, such as ureteric calculus, stricture or tumour, or bladder lesions. A drainage catheter may be left in place at the end of the procedure and follow-up contrast studies may then be carried out to monitor the effects of treatment. Alternatively a stent may be introduced, either percutaneously or using a combined approach via the bladder, so that strictures or tumours may be by-passed to relieve obstruction.

Retrograde pyelography

This procedure has been much less commonly used since antegrade pyelography was introduced; it involves the insertion of a catheter in the ureter via the bladder during cystoscopy. Contrast studies are then carried out. The procedure requires a general anaesthetic, unlike antegrade pyelography.

Micturating cystourethrography

This is usually carried out in infants or children with possible ureteric reflux or urethral valve (male infants). The bladder is catheterised and filled with contrast medium. When micturition commences the catheter is removed and radiographs are obtained of the voiding bladder and of the urethra. The ureteric regions are examined for evidence of reflux. The procedure is carried out under fluoroscopic control and because of the proximity of the area of interest to the gonads the radiation dose is relatively high unless the duration of fluoroscopy is kept to a minimum. An alternative technique has been developed to reduce the radiation burden – direct or indirect radionuclide cystography. This technique is less precise than contrast studies in terms of anatomical resolution, but ureteric reflux is demonstrated very effectively – increasing radioactivity is observed and recorded in the ureteric region(s) during and after micturition. The indirect test resembles excretory urography, in that the dose of radionuclide is administered intravenously. The direct technique uses urethral catherterisation in the same way as micturating cystourethrography.

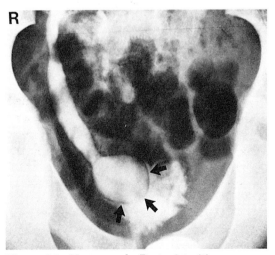

Figure 4.2   Ureterocoele. Post micturition radiograph showing the dilated lower end of the ureter – 'cobra head' appearance. A full bladder may conceal this and the patient may be seen to have only a dilated ureter down to the vesicoureteric junction

It is claimed that the radiation dose is significantly smaller using this latter method and is thus preferable to micturating cystourethrography, in the paediatric age group in particular.

Hysterosalpingography

This is carried out by introducing a contrast agent directly into the uterine cavity and is used to demonstrate anatomical malformations and variants; it is also useful in the investigation of infertility in selected patients. Its usefulness has diminished with the increasing use of ultrasonography and laparoscopic techniques.

Anatomical variants in the genitourinary tract

Because of the complex embryological development and migration of rudimentary precursors of the genitourinary system, and also its differentiation into male and female organs, anatomical variants are relatively common. Some are discovered coincidentally during the investigation of unrelated systems and symptoms. Others are undoubtedly associated with symptoms. For example, duplex kidneys may be discovered incidentally; horseshoe kidneys predispose to infections. The following conditions are fairly common:

- duplex kidney with double ureters, which may or may not unite before joining the bladder; ureterocele may be an associated feature (Fig. 4.2);
- ectopic kidney, usually lying in the pelvis;
- crossed fusion of a kidney; the 'crossed' kidney has a ureter that enters the bladder on its correct side;
- horseshoe kidney (Fig. 4.3);
- ectopic ureteric insertion, usually associated with a duplex system; for example the ureter may enter the vagina, causing incontinence and urinary dribbling;
- fistulae, usually between the bladder and rectum in anorectal agenesis ('imperforate anus');

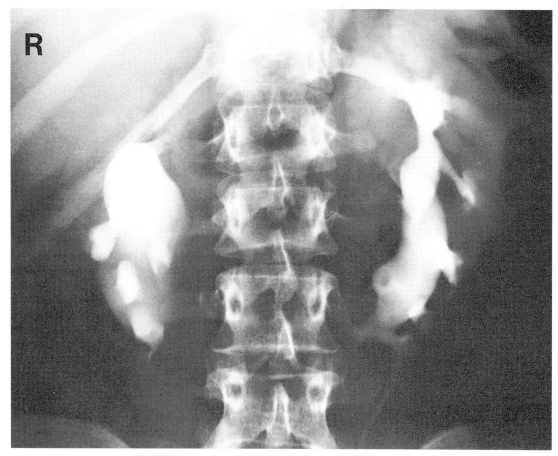

Figure 4.3   Horseshoe kidney. Abnormal axis of the kidneys with some of the calyces pointing medially. The soft tissue bridge between the two lower poles may cause ureteric compression resulting in hydronephrosis

- urethral valves and diverticula;
- hypospadias and ambiguous genitalia;
- bicornuate uterus (Fig. 4.4); other more complex forms of duplicity of the uterus and vagina are also described but are rare.

Radiological investigation of common urinary tract problems

Symptoms and signs originating in the urinary tract are relatively common in all age groups, but particularly in the paediatric age group and in the elderly. The most appropriate use of imaging techniques and the main radiological features of these disorders are outlined here.

Renal colic

Excretory urography should be performed during or soon after the episode. Oedema of the ureteric orifice after the passage of a small calculus may cause distension of the lower ureter. An opaque calculus may be visible on the control abdominal radiograph. Signs of obstruction include a delayed 'nephrogram' (opacification of the renal parenchyma by contrast medium) on the affected side, and dilatation of the collecting system and ureter as far distally as the point of obstruction (Fig. 4.1). In severe cases the system may leak spontaneously, causing extravasation of urine and contrast medium into the soft tissues surrounding the kidney and ureter.

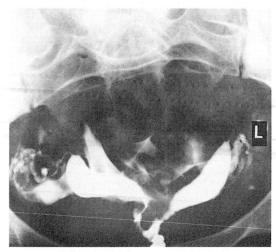

Figure 4.4   Hysterosalpingogram showing a bicornuate uterus with two separate cervical canals and uterine bodies. The fallopian tubes are patent – free peritoneal spill of contrast is shown on both sides

Renal failure

Ultrasonography is the best investigation in this situation because it is possible to assess renal size and shape and parenchymal thickness without the need for contrast agents. In chronic renal failure the kidneys may be small and contain more echoes than usual (echogenic kidney). Alternatively the kidneys may be enlarged – acutely in renal venous thrombosis and chronically in polycystic kidneys. Post-renal obstruction causing renal failure can also be detected by ultrasonography; here both ureters are usually obstructed, either by retroperitoneal disease, e.g. retroperitoneal fibrosis, or by bladder or other pelvic disease, such as an advanced infiltrating tumour.

Renal mass

The patient may present with haematuria, a palpable abdominal mass, evidence of widespread tumour dissemination, or the renal tumour may be detected as a coincidental finding. Simple renal cysts are relatively common and do not usually justify further investigation (Fig. 4.5). Ultrasonography helps to distinguish between a cystic and a solid mass. Complex sonographic patterns usually indicate a malignant tumour and further radiological investigations are indicated to assess the lesion in terms of local spread and invasion of adjacent structures, and to assess evidence of metastatic spread (Fig. 4.6).

Renal tract injury

The main indication for excretion urography in trauma is to assess the presence and function of the contralateral (hopefully uninjured) kidney, particularly if surgery on the injured kidney is being considered. Trauma to the bladder or urethra is generally associated with pelvic fractures. Non-function of the traumatised kidney on excretion urography may indicate damage to the renal artery. Extravasation of contrast medium may occur if there is a tear in the renal cortex and capsule or if the ureter is avulsed. The bladder may be displaced or compressed by pelvic haematoma. Ascending urethrography is occasionally used to assess urethral injuries.

Hypertension

Many renal disorders are associated with hypertension, e.g. chronic pyelonephritis or glomerulonephritis, polycystic kidneys, renal

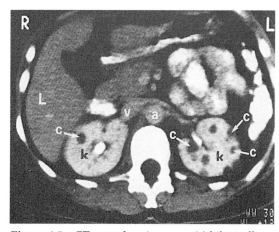

Figure 4.5   CT scan showing cysts (c) bilaterally in the kidneys (k). The left renal vein passes anterior to the aorta (a) and enters the inferior vena cava (v). The liver (L) is also demonstrated

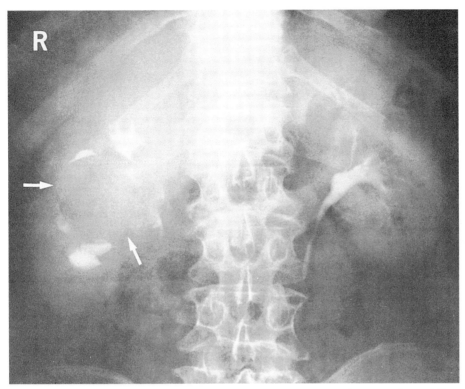

Figure 4.6a   Intravenous pyelogram showing a space occupying lesion in the middle of the right kidney – the pelvicalyceal system is compressed and displaced by the mass

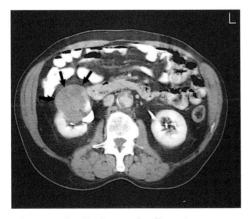

Figure 4.6b   Right renal cell carcinoma (arrowed) demonstrated by CT

artery stenosis (Fig. 4.7) and renal papillary necrosis. Ultrasonography is the best initial investigation and may give enough relevant information so that no other radiological technique may be necessary. A variety of signs may be detected, depending on the nature of the underlying renal disease – small scarred kidneys in chronic pyelonephritis, and large kidneys with numerous cystic masses in polycystic kidneys. In renal artery stenosis the affected kidney may be smaller than its partner; a difference of up to 2 cm is a normal variation in adults but a discrepancy of more than 2 cm is regarded as significant. Radionuclide renography is a sensitive indicator of renal artery stenosis, showing the discrepancy in size and excretion rate between the two kidneys. Selective renal angiography confirms the presence of a stenosis and angioplasty may be attempted during the same procedure (Fig. 4.7).

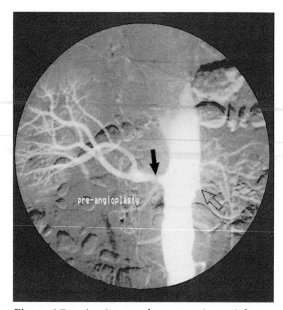

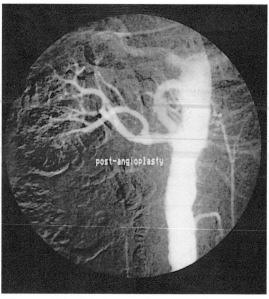

Figure 4.7a   Angiogram demonstrating a tight stenosis just beyond the origin of the right renal artery (arrow). The left renal artery is occluded (open arrow)

Figure 4.7b   Following balloon angioplasty the right renal artery stenosis has been successfully dilated

Endocrine disorders

Examples of endocrine disorders where lesions may be found in close proximity to the kidneys include phaeochromocytoma, Cushing's syndrome and Conn's syndrome (hyper-aldosteronism). There are specific clinical and biochemical indicators in these disorders but radiological investigations – CT and MRI in particular – are used to investigate these adrenal-based disorders. Some specific radionuclide studies may be carried out and venous sampling of the blood draining from the gland and its lesion, or ectopic lesions, may be carried out under fluoroscopic control. In the paediatric group it may be difficult to distinguish between primary renal or adrenal (or neurogenic) tumours and multiple imaging procedures may be necessary before surgical resection. Fetal adrenal masses may be detected during obstetric ultrasound monitoring; some of them regress spontaneously but others may need comprehensive radiological assessment in infancy.

Chapter 5

The skeletal system

- The most common indications for obtaining radiographs of the skeletal system are:

  - trauma
  - back pain
  - joint symptoms – pain, stiffness, swelling.

- Congenital skeletal anomalies and variants are relatively common and should not be mistaken for acquired disease. These variants are usually discovered coincidentally and almost never cause symptoms.

- Some skeletal disorders do not produce radiographically detectable abnormalities early in their course and this may lead to diagnostic errors. This is particularly important in skeletal trauma and in bone infection (osteomyelitis); metastatic deposits from non-skeletal primary tumours may also cause symptoms without producing radiographically detectable bone abnormalities. Specific examples of skeletal trauma and their diagnostic problems are discussed later. In all these situations radionuclide imaging may give important information. Bone-seeking isotopes are concentrated in areas of bone repair where osteoblastic activity is at its most intense. Fractures, infections and even tumours provoke a reparative response and thus, even at an early stage, radionuclide imaging may be positive (localised 'hot spots' of concentrated isotope) when radiographs are negative. This fact has important medicolegal implications, particularly in skeletal trauma.

- Radiographic bone abnormalities fall into a few broad descriptive categories. Bone is either destroyed (lysis) or laid down (sclerosis). The former causes loss of bone density and the latter results in increased bone density. The underlying pathological process may nevertheless be very different. Many disorders cause a combination of the two processes, giving a 'mixed' radiographic picture. In view of this apparent limited range of radiographic abnormalities, many other factors are taken into account when the diagnosis is made – the extent of skeletal involvement, associated joint or soft tissue signs, the age of the patient, etc.

- Many disorders affecting the skeleton cause widespread loss of bone density – osteopenia or osteoporosis. The severity of the demineralisation is difficult to assess from plain radiographs except in extreme cases, and several alternative methods of measuring bone density are in common use. Biochemical assessment of bone metabolism, especially calcium, phosphate and alkaline phosphatase levels, are also important diagnostic aids. In several conditions, such as osteomalacia and hyperparathyroidism, they are much more sensitive than radiographic assessment. It is important to correlate clinical, radiological, biochemical and haematological findings in all complex bone disorders. If bone biopsy becomes an important element of the diagnostic process, this can be carried out under radiological control – fluoroscopy or CT.

- Not all bone disorders arise primarily in the skeleton; there are many systemic or multisystem disorders that affect bone maturation and metabolism. Likewise, joint symptoms may be a manifestation of a variety of non-articular disorders.

Growth and development of the skeleton

- Calcification and ossification of the underlying osteoid matrix and cartilage occurs in a predictable progression throughout intrauterine life and during infancy and childhood. The skeleton becomes fully mature between 16 and 18 years of age, when longitudinal bone growth ceases. Using plain radiography the skeleton can be 'aged' on the basis of the pattern of ossification of the skeleton; radiographs of the non-dominant hand and wrist allow accurate assessments of bone age to be made between the ages of 18 months and complete skeletal maturation. In infancy, radiographs of the knees and feet are particularly useful for 'dating' some of the earliest epiphyses to ossify.
- This maturation process may be affected in several ways, either by specific bone disorders or by systemic or generalised disease. Inherited disorders, such as some of the chromosomal syndromes, also affect skeletal development. The radiographic pattern of abnormal development is often distinctive and diagnostic, although radiographic skeletal surveys deliver a significant dose of radiation to young children and should not be carried out without full consultation.

- Normal bone modelling is dependent on normal physical development – 'floppy' babies tend to have straight spines or to develop abnormal curvatures. Non-weight-bearing affects the development of the pelvis and lower limbs particularly – poor muscle tone or control produces thin 'spindly' and demineralised bones. This occurs in children with severe neurological disorders such as cerebral palsy.
- Bone is a dynamic structure; throughout childhood osteoblastic activity is intense and exceeds osteoclastic activity. This is particularly apparent in radionuclide imaging of the skeleton – the bone ends (i.e. the metaphyses) show intense isotope uptake, often enough to obscure pathological lesions such as osteomyelitis or skeletal injury. Longitudinal bone growth occurs at the metaphysis and periosteal activity along the diaphysis (or shaft) of the bone contributes to circumferential growth.
- Long bones develop from three distinct components: the epiphysis (sub-articular bone ends), the metaphysis, incorporating the epiphyseal plate, and the diaphysis or bone shaft. By the age of 16–18 years virtually all the epiphyses have fused with the diaphyses and longitudinal growth ceases. Bone repair, e.g. after a fracture, then becomes predominantly the function of the periosteum.
- Premature fusion of the epiphyses may occur under certain circumstances – inflammatory joint disorders in childhood and traumatic involvement of the epiphyseal growth plate are examples. Premature fusion results in early cessation of longitudinal growth and there may be generalised short stature if the fusion is caused by multiple affected arthritic joints, or isolated stunted growth in the case of trauma.
- Table 5.1 summarises the most important disorders that affect these key areas of the developing skeleton. Rare inherited disorders (bone dysplasias and chromosomal disorders) cause a variety of specific abnor-

Table 5.1   Disorders affecting growth and development of the skeleton

Site	*Abnormalities and their significance*
● Epiphysis	Delayed development – epiphyses small and fragmented. Inherited dysplasia, but hypothyroidism is an important cause. Long-term complication is premature degenerative change, especially in weight-bearing joints. Bone age assessment often impossible
● Metaphysis	Dysplasias, metabolic disorders, infiltrations, infections. All these may cause significant and possibly permanent impairment of bone growth and development. Inherited deficiency of alkaline phosphatase may cause severe deformities. Acquired rickets on the other hand may be reversed, leading to normal bone development. Trauma (in child abuse) causes microfractures
● Diaphysis	Commonly affected by trauma. Repair process depends on periosteum. Some fractures fail to heal and unite, causing pseudoarthrosis. This is a recogised feature of neurofibromatosis. Stress or fatigue fractures occur in the diaphysis. Transverse or chalk-stick fractures indicate abnormal underlying bone (osteopetrosis, for example). Multiple fractures in osteogenesis imperfecta may cause severe deformities and limb shortening

Table 5.2   Examples of the distribution of lesions in some common skeletal disorders

Disorder	*Distribution*
● Paget's disease (Fig. 5.1)	Skull – may be predominantly lytic lesion but later sclerotic with thickened vault Pelvis – thickened bone with coarse trabecular pattern and increased density Limb bone – subarticular sclerosis and coarse trabeculation extending into diaphysis
● Hyperparathyroidism (Fig. 5.2)	Hands – acro-osteolysis, subperiosteal bone resorption, cartilage calcification, bone cysts Chest – erosion of the lateral ends of the clavicles; generalised abnormality of bone trabeculation Abdomen – nephrocalcinosis
● Osteomalacia (Fig. 5.3)	Looser's zones in clavicles, scapulae, pubic rami Deformed pelvis Bowed lower limbs
● Myelomatosis	Skull – multiple lytic lesions Chest – expanding rib lesions Spine – osteopenia, collapsed vertebrae Limbs – endosteal erosion due to intramedullary expanding lesions

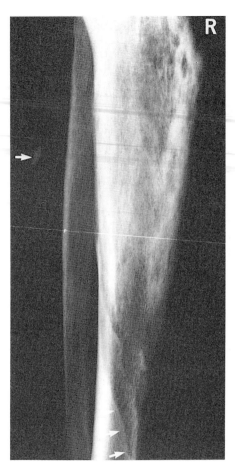

Figure 5.1   Paget's disease affecting upper end of the tibia. Characteristic 'flame' shaped appearance at lower end. Coincidental calcification in soft tissues – due to cysticercosis

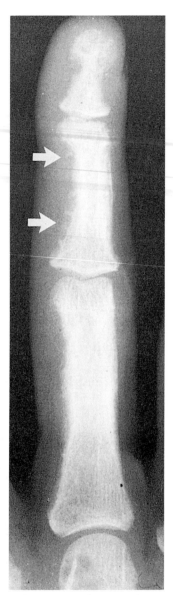

Figure 5.2   Hyperparathyroidism. Subperiosteal bone resorption shown in the phalanges, with resorption of the tuft of the terminal phalanx

Table 5.3 Locally destructive bone lesions

Causes	Radiological features
● Well-defined margins	
e.g. bone 'cysts'	Often detected in childhood
	Humerus – present with pathological fracture
fibrous cortical defects	Superficial lesions; no significance; usually disappear
enchondroma	Hands; may have flecks of calcification
eosinophil granuloma	Skull and elsewhere, solitary or multiple
sarcoidosis (Fig. 5.4)	Hands; associated soft tissue swelling

Note: Some of these lesions may be discovered coincidentally, and there is some overlap in the radiological appearances. The site of the lesion is important in determining the likely diagnosis

● Poorly defined margins	
e.g. metastases, myelomatosis	Multiple, variable appearance but may be solitary initially
primary bone tumours	Localised but variable soft tissue extension
infection (Fig. 5.5)	Osteomyelitis tends to occur at ends of bones in the young, but there may be predisposing circumstances – trauma, diabetes, surgery, etc.

Note: Considerable overlap in radiological signs. Skeletal survey, radionuclide studies, and bone biopsy may be necessary to resolve the problem

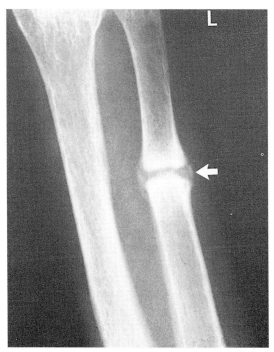

Figure 5.3 Osteomalacia. Characteristic Looser's zone in shaft of ulna

malities at one or more sites (a combination of epiphyseal and metaphyseal abnormalities, for example). These may result in severe growth retardation and dwarfism. A radiographic survey of the skeleton is an important part of the genetic assessment and counselling process in these circumstances.

Analysing radiographic abnormalities in the skeleton

● Fractures and their consequences – displacement, angulation, healing, non-union and evidence of surgical intervention – form a well-defined group of radiological appearances. Trauma to joints – dislocations, associated bony injuries – also give characteristic signs. It is important to rule out an underlying bone lesion or a generalised abnormality that predisposes to fractures.

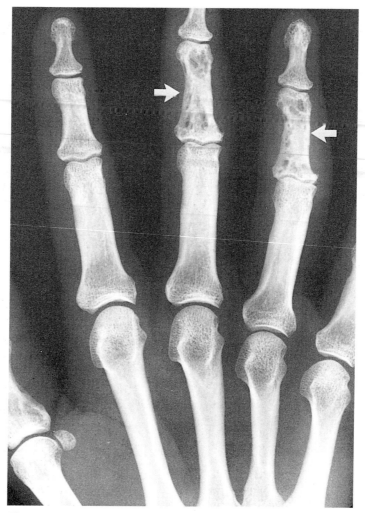

Figure 5.4   Sarcoidosis. Small well-defined 'cysts' shown in the phalanges. When skeletal changes occur in sarcoidosis they are generally associated with skin lesions

● Non-traumatic disorders of the skeleton require a more systematic approach, involving the following stages.

  – Identification of the type of lesion – destructive, sclerotic, localised or widespread, involving joints and/or soft tissues.
  – Assessment of the full extent of the lesion(s). This may eventually require the use of other imaging techniques such as CT or MRI.

  – Determination of the extent of the abnormality in the skeleton as a whole and whether any lesion may be accessible for biopsy.
  – Consideration of the general health of the patient, the mode of presentation, the patient's age, evidence of systemic ill health. The differential diagnosis in cases where a tumour is being considered depends to a large extent on the patient's age. Childhood tumours such as Ewing's sarcoma may resemble

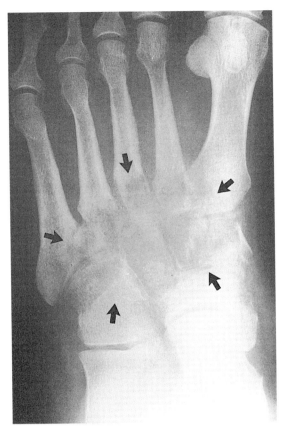

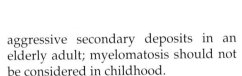

Figure 5.5   Tuberculous infection. Ill-defined area of bone destruction affecting the distal tarsus and proximal metatarsals. No periosteal reaction, which would be evident in pyogenic infection

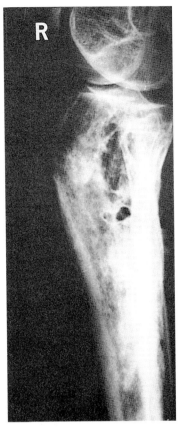

Figure 5.6   Chronic osteomyelitis – upper end of tibia. Abnormal bone texture with areas of increased and decreased density, cortical thickening and irregularity

aggressive secondary deposits in an elderly adult; myelomatosis should not be considered in childhood.

- Some bone lesions have very characteristic appearances, e.g. rickets, and little or no corroborative radiological evidence is necessary. Conversely, acroosteolysis (dissolution of the tufts of the terminal phalanges) occurs in a variety of conditions and full clinical and biochemical assessment is necessary.
- Evidence of growth retardation with specific clinical features (e.g. abnormal facial appearance, low-set ears, supernumerary teeth, poly- or syndactyly) are very suggestive of a dysplastic or dysmorphic syndrome and full clinical, radiological, biochemical and genetic assessment is usually carried out.

This is not an exhaustive list but it illustrates the important elements of the analysis of radiographic bone or joint abnormalities. The 'geographical' distribution of the lesion(s) in the skeleton as a whole is a useful discriminator.

When planning further radiographic assessment, Table 5.2 illustrates some of the most common sites of involvement in a few wellknown skeletal disorders.

Table 5.4 Locally sclerotic lesions

Causes	Radiological features
● Anatomical variants e.g. 'bone islands'	Incidental finding – pelvis, femora mainly
● Degenerative joint disease	Osteophytes may produce localised sclerosis around joints
● Infection (Fig. 5.6)	Chronic osteomyelitis. Mixed pattern of lysis and sclerosis, periosteal new bone, deformity
● Tumours	
e.g. benign osteoma	Skull, very dense
osteoid osteoma	Usually limb bone, child or adolescent, pain (nocturnal). Intense sclerosis if sited in or near cortex
osteogenic sarcoma (Fig. 5.7)	Characteristic bone-forming tumour with extension into soft tissues and intense periosteal response
lymphoma	May cause 'ivory vertebra'. Usually mixed lesion
metastasis (Fig. 5.8)	Usually multiple but may be solitary. Prostate and breast are most common sources
● Miscellaneous disorders e.g. bone infarct	Osteonecrosis, e.g. in divers. Usually medullary, long bones. Geographical area of increased density
Paget's disease (Fig. 5.1)	Skull, pelvis, etc. Thickened bone with coarse trabecular pattern
trauma	Healing fractures or stress fractures may produce localised sclerosis with no visible fracture line
post-radiotherapy	Form of osteonecrosis, e.g. ribs after breast cancer treatment

Types of bone abnormality

It is convenient to classify bone lesions along the following lines to arrive at a reasonable list of differential diagnoses:

● locally   destructive   (e.g.   infections, tumours)
● locally sclerotic (e.g. chronic infection, some tumours, avascular necrosis)
● widespread loss of density (e.g. osteoporosis, metabolic bone disorders, e.g. hyperparathyroidism, steroid therapy)
● widespread increased density (e.g. some metastatic tumours, myelofibrosis, fluorosis)
● mixed lesions (e.g. Paget's disease, chronic infection)
● bone growth and modelling abnormalities (e.g. bone dysplasias, neurofibromatosis, trauma)

● primary joint disease affecting adjacent bony structures (e.g. inflammatory joint disease, some synovial tumours)
● soft tissue disorders that affect joints (e.g. collagen diseases, soft tissue tumours or infections that invade or compress adjoining bone)
● miscellaneous radiological features (e.g. periosteal reaction, intra-articular calcification, soft-tissue calcification).

Tables 5.3–5.6 summarise the most important radiological features of these disorders.

Skeletal trauma

● Radiographs are used to confirm or exclude fractures, to assess the type and complexity of a fracture and the relationship of bony fragments to each other and

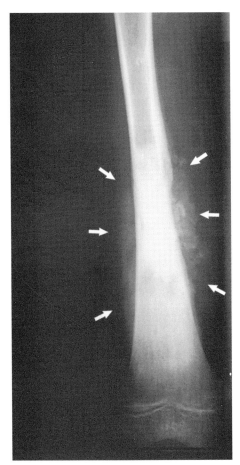

Figure 5.7 Radiograph of the right femur showing an osteogenic sarcoma. Young patient, male. Note unfused epiphyses. Irregular bone texture with a mass extending into the soft tissues; marked periosteal new bone formation

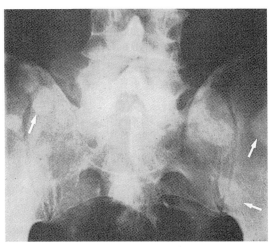

Figure 5.8 Sclerotic metastases in the lumbar spine and pelvis from carcinoma of the prostate

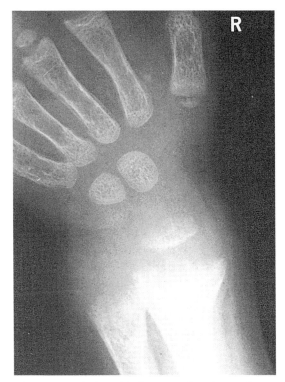

Figure 5.9 Rickets. Right wrist. Cupping and splaying of metaphyses at lower end of radius and ulna. Bones generally demineralised, periosteal reaction shown in long bones

Table 5.5   Widespread loss of bone density

Causes	Radiological features
● Osteoporosis e.g. 'senile' or post-menopausal disuse adjoning inflammation steroid therapy	All these conditions produce bone demineralisation, and this may predispose to vertebral collapse, rib fractures; densitometry assessment more accurate than radiographs
● Metabolic bone disease e.g. osteomalacia, rickets hyperparathyroidism (Figs 5.2, 5.3, 5.9)	These disorders produce characteristic radiological signs, but the predominating feature may be generalised demineralisation of the skeleton Osteomalacia – pseudo-fractures, deformities Hyperparathyroidism – bone cysts, sub-periosteal bone resorption, acro-osteolysis, nephrocalcinosis, soft-tissue (articular) calcification Rickets – characteristic flaring, splaying and irregularity of the metaphyses in the growing skeleton. Wide zone of unossified matrix
● Infiltration e.g. metastases myelomatosis leukaemia	Diffuse demineralisation may occur without identifiable localised bone destruction
● Haemolytic disorders e.g. thalassaemia	Marrow overactivity and overgrowth giving characteristic appearances in the small bones of the hand particularly

Table 5.6   Widespread increase in bone density

Causes	Radiological features
● Congenital – osteopetrosis	Rare conditions resulting in characteristic sclerosis of the skeleton and bone fragility resulting in 'chalk-stick' fractures. 'Marble-bone' disease in its severest form is lethal. Bands or islands of very dense bone affecting all bones
● Acquired e.g. metastases	Usually from prostate or breast. May coalesce to produce dense skeleton
myelofibrosis	Uniformly dense bones. Splenomegaly. Several causes including drug-induced myelosclerosis
fluorosis	Endemic areas, e.g. Middle East. Accompanied by soft tissue (ligamentous) ossification
sickle-cell disease	Generalised increased density with localised areas of bone infarction, e.g. humeral heads, vertebrae

(a)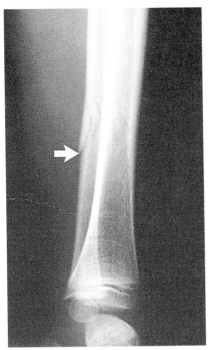

(b)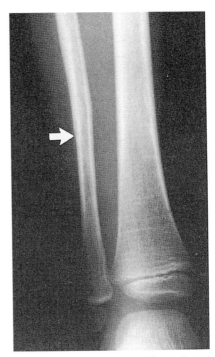

Figure 5.10 *(a)* Spiral fracture through shaft of fibula. The fracture line is only visible on the lateral view. *(b)* The AP view could be considered normal. This illustrates the value of obtaining two views at right angles in cases of skeletal trauma

to adjoining structures, and to show possible underlying predisposing conditions such as metastatic deposits. Radiographs are also useful in the follow-up of fractures to show healing (or lack of it) and resultant deformity or other complications, e.g. infection.

- Similarly, dislocations of joints, even in the absence of a fracture, can be assessed radiographically. Here some additional alternative projections may be necessary, e.g. axial view of the shoulder joint.
- The golden rule of radiography in skeletal trauma is that views in two planes must be obtained to confirm or exclude a fracture, because a fracture line or a deformity may only be visible in one plane (Fig. 5.10).
- Transverse (or chalk-stick) fractures of the shafts of long bones usually indicate underlying bone pathology, e.g. Paget's disease or one of the disorders giving rise to 'brittle bones', e.g. osteopetrosis.

- Stress or fatigue fractures occur in active individuals, e.g. athletes, and the sites depend on the activity. For example, long distance runners develop undisplaced, incomplete fractures in the upper third of the tibia (Fig. 5.11) or in the metatarsals. They are painful and appear as localised areas of increased density on radiographs, with some periosteal reaction and surrounding soft tissue calcification (callus). Paget's disease also predisposes to incomplete or stress fractures (Fig. 5.12).
- Ambulant and adventurous young children often sustain long-bone (usually mid-shaft) fractures, but in non-accidental injury, usually occurring in infancy, fractures occur in unusual sites, e.g. posterior ends of the ribs, scapulae, hand and foot bones, and metaphyses (Fig. 5.13). Fractures may be multiple and of different ages and stages of repair. The ageing of these fractures is often imprecise because

(a)   (b)

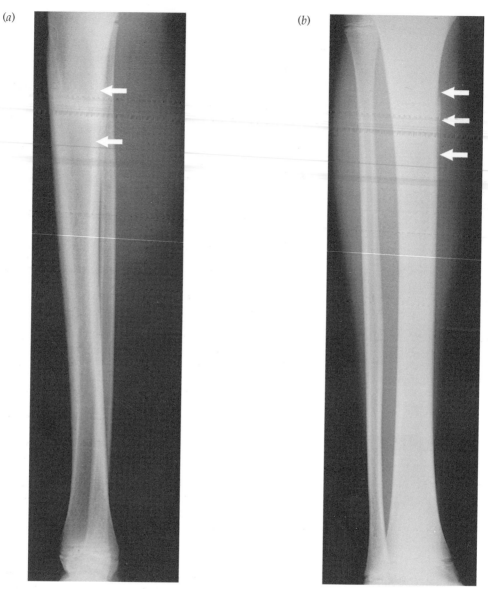

Figure 5.11   AP and lateral projections showing a stress fracture of the tibia – area of sclerosis and periosteal reaction. Young athlete

Table 5.7 Common joint disorders

Causes	Radiological features
● Osteoarthritis	● Narrowed joint space, marginal osteophytes, surrounding sclerosis, subchondral cysts Affects spine, hips, knees mainly; also hands – distal interphalangeal joints and first metacarpophalangeal joints in particular
● Rheumatoid arthritis (RA) and Still's disease (juvenile chronic arthritis) (Fig. 5.18)	● Erosive arthropathy, symmetrical involvement usually. Proximal interphalangeal, metacarpo- and metatarsophalangeal joints commonly Acute phase – soft-tissue swelling, periarticular osteoporosis. Cortical erosions Later – joint subluxation, 'arthritis mutilans' Juvenile form – few, if any, erosions; soft-tissue swelling and hyperaemia leading to epiphyseal overgrowth followed by premature fusion
● Gout (Fig. 5.19)	● Erosions affecting mainly the interphalangeal joints. Deep, punched out, with less surrounding osteoporosis than in RA Crystal deposition in joints (sodium biurate)
● Psoriasis (Fig. 5.20)	● Resembles RA except that distal interphalangeal joints of hands and feet are disproportionately affected Skin disorders may not be severe or even prominent
● Ankylosing spondylitis	● Sacroiliitis; calcification of longitudinal ligaments to form continuous bridges over discs – 'bamboo spine'. Causes severe kyphosis in later stages Synovial joints also affected by seronegative arthritis similar to RA with severe degenerative changes superimposed
● Haemophilia (Fig. 5.21)	● Knees, ankles, elbows – chronic or repeated haemarthrosis, with changes similar to juvenile arthritis initially, followed by degenerative changes
● Neuropathic joints (Fig. 5.22)	● Impaired sensation (diabetes, syringomyelia) leading to severe degenerative changes and total disruption and dislocation of affected joints (Charcot joints)

of the repetitive nature of the injury. This may account for the abundant amount of callus that forms around the fracture(s) in some cases.

Difficult areas in skeletal trauma

Undiagnosed fractures and dislocations can have serious medical and legal consequences and may result in severe deformity and disability. Examples include the following.

● Undiagnosed scaphoid fracture: causes chronic pain and may result in osteonecrosis of the bone.

● Fractures of the femoral neck may be impacted, with no apparent fracture line radiographically and no deformity (Fig. 5.14). In this circumstance an MRI scan may be diagnostic (Fig. 5.15). Avascular necrosis of the femoral head is a recognised complication and may necessitate prosthetic replacement of the hip joint.

● Posterior dislocation of the shoulder or hip joints may not be apparent on standard radiographs and additional projections are necessary for confirmation. Unsuspected fractures of the humeral and femoral heads may be discovered in association with these dislocations.

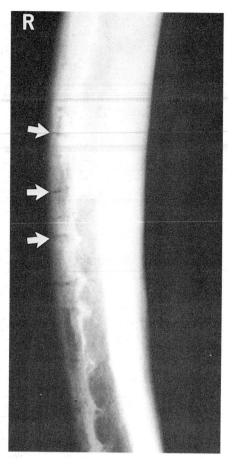

Figure 5.12 'Stress' fractures seen on the convex surface of the bowed femur in a patient with Paget's disease. A pathological transverse fracture may occur through this brittle bone

- Complex fracture/dislocations of the wrist, foot and ankle, e.g. translunar dislocation, require radiographs in at least two planes for complete assessment (Fig. 5.16). There are usually associated relatively unimpressive fractures, e.g. of the radial and ulnar styloid processes, which are easily overlooked. Avascular necrosis of bone is a serious long-term complication of many complex fractures, resulting in severe mechanical instability of joints, pain and disability.

- Skull fractures and spinal fractures give rise to diagnostic difficulties and are discussed in Chapter 6.

Use of alternative imaging techniques in the skeleton

It will be apparent that in some circumstances plain radiographs of the skeleton are inadequate for the assessment of early phases of damage and repair, whether the cause is trauma, infection or even tumour. In this situation radionuclide studies are very useful because they are more sensitive to increased osteoblastic activity than radiographs. Therefore this technique has become well established in the early detection of bone disease (Fig. 5.17) and is particularly useful where the possible complications of that disease are to be avoided. In possible avascular necrosis of bone, 'cold' areas on radionuclide scanning confirm the diagnosis, e.g. in the femoral head following a fracture of the neck.

MRI has also become established as an important and sensitive technique for the early detection of bone marrow disease and soft tissue abnormalities adjacent to bone or within joints. Cancellous bone is not visible on MRI scans but the consequences of bone trauma are frequently visible, e.g. paraspinal masses, disruption of joint structures.

Radiology of joint diseases

- On clinical grounds alone it may be difficult to distinguish between the different forms of arthritis, although the predominant site of pain and stiffness and the distribution of affected joints may give some indication of the likely diagnosis.
- It must be remembered that 'arthralgia' is a fairly common accompaniment of a variety of non-articular, systemic disorders. A complete assessment of the clinical history and examination is necessary; other non-radiological investigations may give strong clues as to the likely diagnosis.

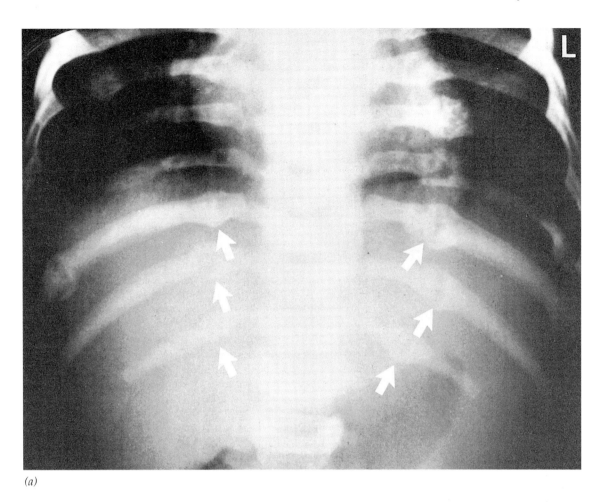

(a)

(b)

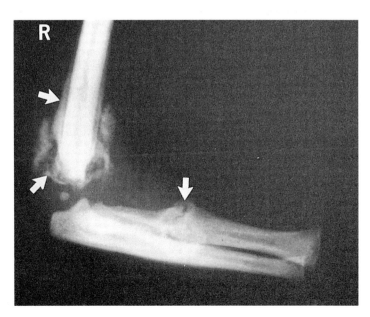

Figure 5.13 *(a)* Non-accidental injury in young child. Numerous fractures at various sites including ribs. *(b)* Same child also has a fracture through the shaft of radius. Calcified subperiosteal haematoma at the lower end of the humerus associated with injury to the metaphysis in this region

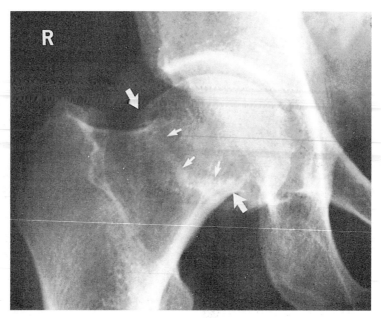

Figure 5.14   Impacted fracture of femoral neck. The dense line (arrowed) indicates the fracture site. This type of fracture is not uncommon in elderly postmenopausal females

- The most common form of joint disease is osteoarthritis (or osteoarthrosis), which is a degenerative process. It affects mainly the weight-bearing joints and is due to general wear and tear. Some occupations involving strenuous manual work (e.g. the use of vibrating tools) may predispose to degeneration. Joint disease from an early age and internal mechanical disruption of joints (e.g. following Perthes' disease) also predispose to premature degenerative change.

- Inflammatory joint disease is relatively common; there are numerous variants that mimic rheumatoid arthritis and there are several types that are seronegative but may be an integral part of systemic or multisystem disease. Some are linked with deposition of crystals or haemosiderin in the joints and form part of a metabolic or haematological disorder. The association between inflammatory bowel disease and

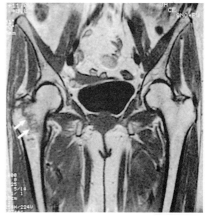

Figure 5.15   MRI scan showing an inter-trochanteric fracture of the right hip (arrowed). There was no plain film evidence of a fracture

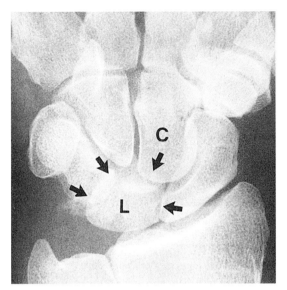

Figure 5.16a Lunate dislocation, wrist AP view, showing the abnormal shape of lunate (L) which appears triangular instead of quadrilateral, and loss of 'joint space'

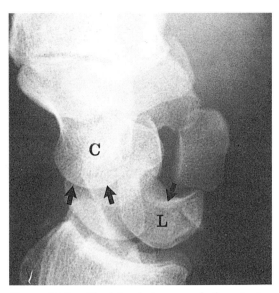

Figure 5.16b The lateral view reveals the extent of injury, showing the dislocation of the lunate. Normally the capitate (C) sits in the concavity of the lunate (L)

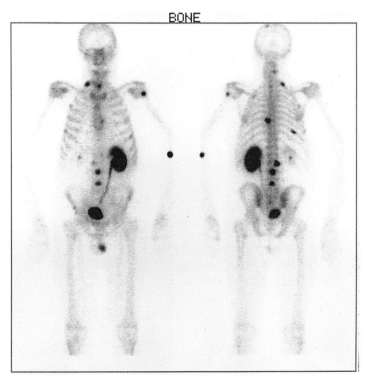

Figure 5.17 Isotope bone scan showing multiple areas of increased uptake ('hot spots') in a patient with prostatic carcinoma with metastases. Note the hydronephrotic obstructed left kidney

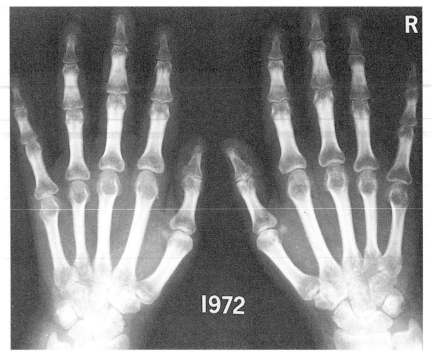

Figure 5.18a   Rheumatoid arthritis showing progression of disease. Initially periarticular osteoporosis and soft tissue swelling; no actual erosions seen

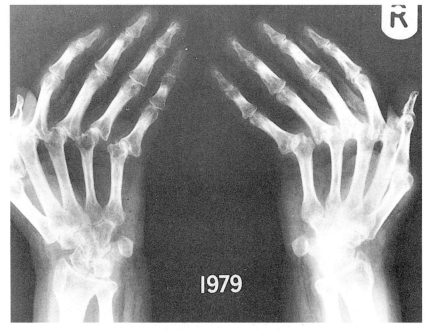

Figure 5.18b   Oblique view of same patient. With time, marked erosive changes occur predominantly affecting the metacarpophalangeal regions which are partially subluxed – the fingers exhibiting ulnar deviation

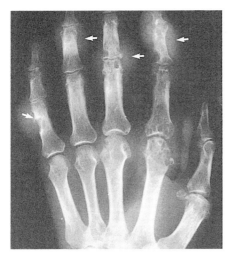

Figure 5.19 Gout – deep erosions with 'overhanging' edges. Associated with eccentric soft tissue swellings

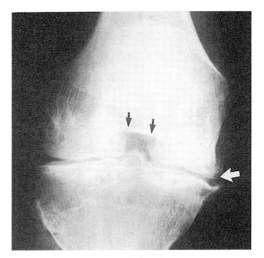

Figure 5.21 Haemophilia. Premature degenerative changes with irregularity of the articular surfaces, squaring of the intercondylar notch and subcortical cyst formation

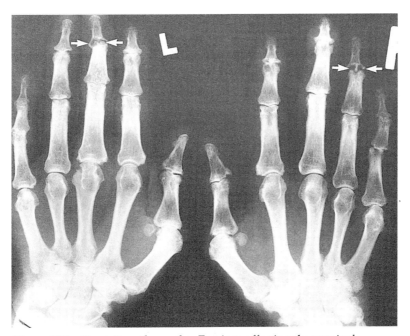

Figure 5.20 Psoriatic arthropathy. Erosions affecting the terminal interphalangeal joints are characteristic of this condition

ankylosing spondylitis and sacroiliitis is well recognised, as is the association between psoriasis and a seronegative erosive arthritis.

- The radiological features of joint disorders can be categorised into:

  - non-specific: signs of effusion
    degenerative osteophytes
    joint space narrowing
    sub-chrondral 'cysts'
  - specific: erosions
    cartilage calcification
    soft-tissue swelling
    periarticular osteoporosis
    long-term complications such as ankylosis, arthritis mutilans and osteonecrosis.

The radiological features of some of the most common forms of arthritis are summarised in Table 5.7.

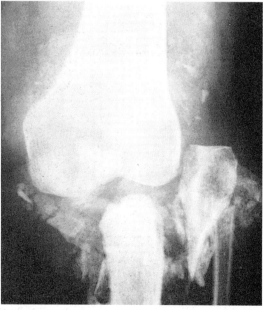

Figure 5.22 Neuropathic joint – left knee. Markedly disorganized with extensive surrounding soft tissue calcification

Miscellaenous signs of bone and joint disease

Periosteal reaction

This has been mentioned several times in this chapter because it is a common accompaniment of bone and joint disease. Periosteal new bone is a reparative response along the shafts of bones and is stimulated by trauma, inflammation, infection and tumours. It causes localised increased density of bone and may produce one of several distinctive radiological patterns – 'lamellar', 'onion skin', 'spiculated', etc., and some of these signs have been attributed to specific disorders. It may occur in response to soft tissue inflammation or infection alongside bone and need not therefore signify a primary bone disorder. One very distinctive pattern is seen in patients with certain lung disorders, e.g. carcinoma – hypertrophic pulmonary osteoarthropathy (HPOA), which is a symmetrical periosteal reaction along the femora, tibiae and forearm bones and is associated with severe, constant pain (Fig. 5.23). The aetiology is not known.

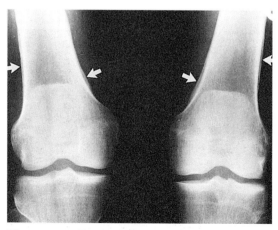

Figure 5.23 Hypertrophic pulmonary osteoarthropathy. Periosteal reaction at the lower ends of both femora in a patient with carcinoma of the lung

Avascular necrosis of bone

This process may be provoked by trauma (resulting in non-union of fractures, e.g. of the scaphoid, femoral head, or talus), barotrauma, ischaemia due to abnormal coagulation in sickle cell disease, or drug therapy, e.g. corticosteroids. The process is not well understood but causes non-uptake of bone-seeking radionuclides, causing 'cold' areas in scans. Perthes' disease is a very specific form of this disorder and occurs in children, usually in boys between the ages of 5 and 8 years (Fig. 5.24). The femoral capital epiphyses become fragmented and small, and later dense. They reform with appropriate therapy (mainly immobilisation) but are usually abnormal in shape and may predispose to premature osteoarthritis. The sclerosis seen in avascular necrosis is due to thickened trabeculae and is attributed to bone repair.

Intra-articular calcification

Degenerative change (osteoarthritis) is associated with calcification of joint fibrocartilage, but cartilage calcification is a prominent feature of pseudo-gout (a crystal deposition arthritis) and metabolic conditions such as hyperparathyroidism, haemochromatosis and ochronosis (Fig. 5.25).

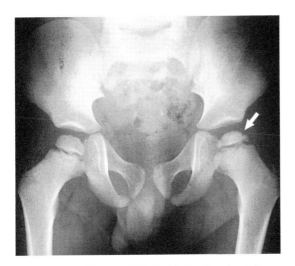

Figure 5.24 Young child. Perthe's disease of the left hip. Note the sclerosis, loss of height and early fragmentation of the capital epiphysis of the left femur (arrowed)

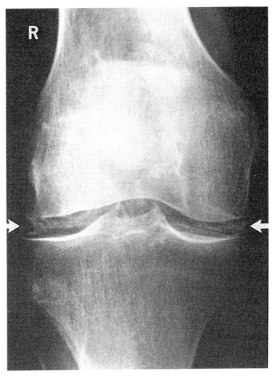

Figure 5.25 Chondrocalcinosis

Soft-tissue calcification around joints

Systemic sclerosis (scleroderma) causes calcification in soft tissues related to joints and on pressure points, i e. the extensor surfaces of joints (Fig. 5.26). The condition may cause a seronegative arthropathy. Extensive para-articular soft-tissue calcification may occur in paralysed patients and calcium deposition has been seen in patients in renal dialysis, especially around the shoulder joints. These calcifications should not be confused with parasitic calcification, which usually occurs in muscles and is typical of cysticercosis.

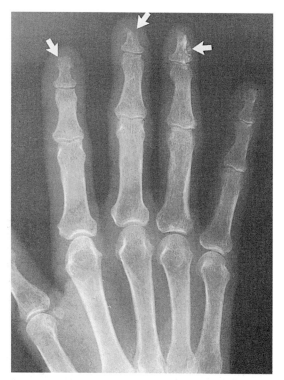

Figure 5.26   Systemic sclerosis. Soft tissue calcification and resorption of tufts of terminal phalanges

Chapter 6

The nervous system

The spine

Plain radiographs of the spine provide information about the shape, size and density of the vertebral bodies and their alignment. Abnormalities associated with congenital and acquired disorders can be shown if there is associated bony involvement, i.e. dumbbell tumour in neurofibromatosis with widening of the neural foramina and erosion of the pedicle (Fig. 6.1).

Changes related to age commence in the spine relatively early in life. Thus spondylosis, a combination of disc degeneration and osteoarthrosis of the posterior spinal joints, is very commonly seen in middle-aged and elderly patients. The intervertebral discs are non-opaque to X-rays so disc herniation cannot be diagnosed on plain radiographs. The sequelae of disc degeneration – adjacent bony sclerosis, osteophyte formation, loss of disc height and osteoarthrosis of the joints of the neural arches can be demonstrated on the plain radiograph.

Any of the generalised disorders affecting the skeleton may also cause changes in the vertebral column. These include Paget's disease, metastases (both lytic and sclerotic) and myeloma (Chapter 5). In addition to these pathological processes, many congenital anatomical variants may affect the spine. Some of these have little clinical significance, e.g. spina bifida occulta. Table 6.1 summarises the radiological abnormalities seen in the spine.

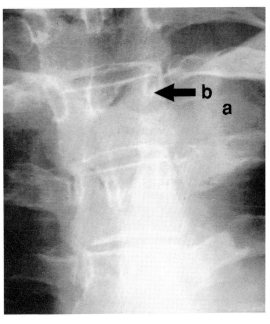

Figure 6.1 Upper thoracic dumbbell tumour with left paravertebral soft tissue mass (a) and erosion of the inferior aspect of the pedicle (b)

Table 6.1   Abnormal appearances in the spine

Causes	*Radiological features*

• Loss of density of vertebral bodies
  With disc space involvement
  infection – pyogenic or
  tuberculous
	Transradiant areas due to bone destruction affecting vertebral bodies on either side of a narrowed disc space. A paraspinal soft tissue mass due to abscess formation may be present and this may calcify later. With healing, fusion of adjacent vertebral bodies often occurs and some deformity results (Fig. 6.2 (a) and (b)

Without disc space involvement metastases, myeloma, osteoporosis	Multiple vertebral bodies may be involved with bony deformity. There may be complete or partial collapse, but the disc spaces are preserved (Figs 6.3 and 6.7)
• Sclerosis of a solitary vertebral body Paget's disease	Affected vertebrae are often enlarged and show either diffuse or marginal 'picture-frame' sclerosis. Other bones may also be involved
Sclerotic metastases, e.g. prostate	May affect only part or whole of vertebra
Lymphoma	Vertebrae tend to be dense. Large para-aortic lymph nodes may erode the anterior surface of the vertebral body, seen on the lateral view
Haemangioma	Normal-sized vertebrae containing dense vertical striations; generally only solitary vertebrae affected

Infection (rare)
    tuberculosis
    toxoplasmosis
    cytomegalic inclusion disease	

Miscellaneous
    hyperparathyroidism
    tuberose sclerosis	

• Neurological disorders
  Congenital
    spina bifida
	Defect in neural arch, widening of interpedicular space, may be associated with a myelomeningocoele

Acquired
    tumour of the spinal canal:
    benign (e.g. neurofibroma,
    meningioma); malignant
    (e.g. metastatic deposit)
	Neurological symptoms due to cord compression. Erosion of pedicles due to local expansion of the tumour or bone destruction may occur

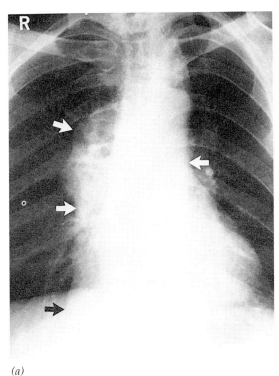

(a)

Figure 6.2   (a) PA chest radiograph of a patient presenting with back pain. Note soft tissue mass (white arrows) extending below the diaphragm (black arrow). (b) Tomographic section of the same patient shows the mass to be paraspinal and associated with a lytic lesion affecting the bodies of T.10/T.11 (black arrows) – there is narrowing of the disc space at this level. These appearances are due to tuberculous infection with an extensive paraspinal abscess, which has caused 'scalloping' of the lateral borders of several thoracic vertebrae

Figure 6.3   Lytic destruction of C.4 and partial collapse of body of C.5 due to metastases from carcinoma of the breast

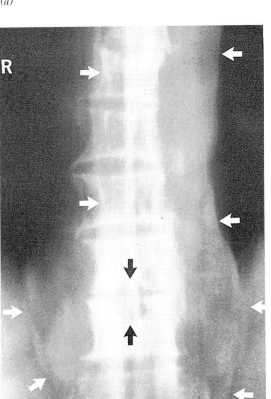

(b)

Miscellaneous causes of back pain

- Defects in the pars interarticularis (spondylolysis) are not uncommon and these may lead to forward slipping of one vertebral body on another (spondylolisthesis) (Fig. 6.4).
- The spine may be affected by many of the erosive arthropathies, e.g. rheumatoid

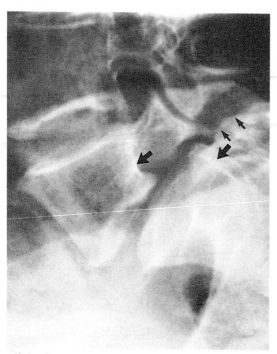

Figure 6.4 Spondylolisthesis at L.5/S.1. The defect in the pars interarticularis at L.5 and the forward slip of L.5 on S.1 is evident

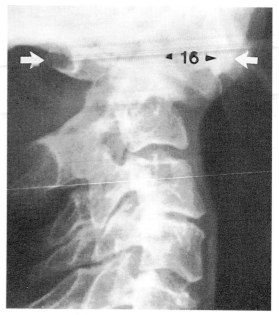

Figure 6.5 Atlantoxial dislocation in a patient with rheumatoid arthritis. Note the position of the anterior arch and the spinous process of the first cervical vertebra in relation to the second. Normally the gap between the anterior arch and odontoid peg should not exceed 3mm

arthritis, Reiter's syndrome, psoriatic arthropathy, etc. The spinal column may eventually become ankylosed.
- Ligamentous degeneration in conditions such as rheumatoid arthritis may lead to dislocation of one vertebra on another, giving rise to long tract signs (Fig. 6.5).

Trauma

Knowledge of the mode of injury is important when assessing patients with spinal trauma. Injury may occur as a result of flexion, extension, rotation or compression, or any combination of these mechanisms. It is important to assess spinal stability on the plain radiograph and early recognition of a fracture/dislocation is of great importance as the onset of neurological signs and symptoms may be delayed. The spine is regarded as a three-column structure: (1) the anterior column – anterior two-thirds of the vertebral bodies; (2) the middle column – posterior one-third of the

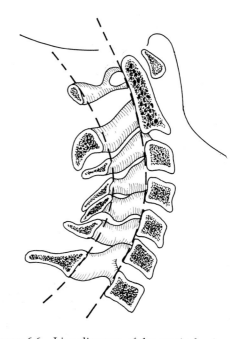

Figure 6.6 Line diagram of the cervical spine. The two lines joining the back of the vertebral bodies and the spinous processes must be in continuity, as shown

vertebral bodies, the articular pillars and the laminae; and (3) the posterior column – the spinous processes. When more than one column is involved in the injury then there is instability (Fig. 6.6). When imaging the cervical spine it is important to ensure the C7–T1 level is included on the lateral view of the cervical spine because up to a third of fractures occur at this level.

Minimal trauma may result in wedge or compression fractures when the bones are abnormal, e.g. osteoporosis, myeloma (Fig. 6.7).

CT is necessary to assess complex fracture/dislocation; it will demonstrate the extent of the injury and the involvement of the spinal canal, and indicate cord or thecal compression (Fig. 6.8).

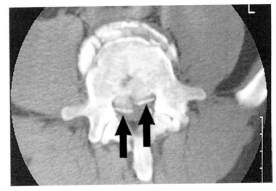

Figure 6.8 Axial CT scan of L5 showing a 'burst' fracture with displacement of bone posteriorly into the spinal canal (arrows) compressing the theca

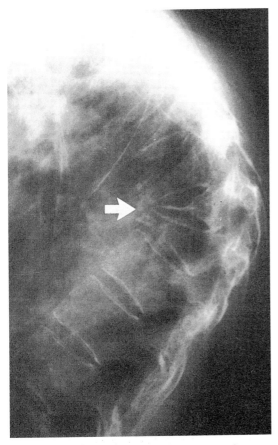

Figure 6.7 Elderly female with osteoporosis. Wedge-shaped collapse of mid-thoracic vertebrae leading to a marked angular kyphosis

Spinal canal and cord lesions

MRI may be helpful when the neurological deficit cannot be explained by plain radiography or CT, or if there is neurological deterioration. MRI is performed to evaluate the structures contained within the spinal canal.

When intrinsic lesions of the spinal cord (Fig. 6.9), or compression of the spinal cord or nerve roots from lesions of the surrounding bones, intervertebral discs (Fig. 6.10) or paravertebral soft tissues are suspected clinically, MRI is the investigation of choice. In some clinical situations, e.g. brachial neuralgia, or when MRI is contraindicated, myelography is still performed, often in combination with CT (Fig. 6.11).

(a)   *(b)*

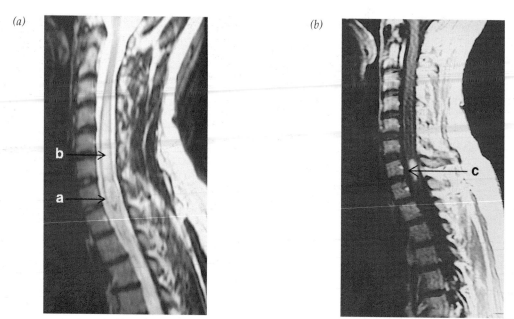

Figure 6.9   *(a)* T2W sagittal MR scan of an intrinsic cord tumour at C7 (a) with extensive abnormal high signal from C3 to C7 which represents fluid within a tumour syrinx (b). *(b)* T1W sagittal enhanced MR scan demonstrating enhancement within the tumour (c)

(a)   *(b)*

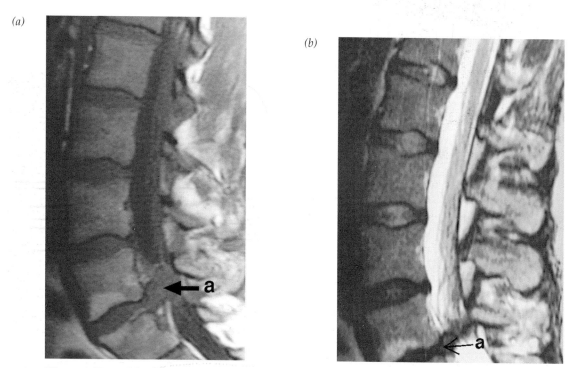

Figure 6.10a and b   T1W sagittal and T2W sagittal MR scans of a large L5-S1 disc herniation (a)

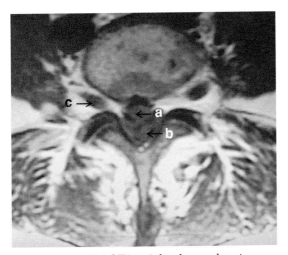

Figure 6.10c Axial T1 weighted scan showing significant thecal compression (b) due to the large central disc herniation. This patient presented with cauda equina symptoms. The L5 nerve root can be seen surrounded by fat beyond the neural foramina (c)

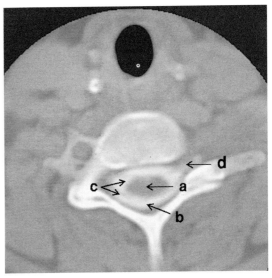

Figure 6.11 Axial CT scan of the cervical spine following myelography. The cervical cord (a) is surrounded by CSF (b) which appears white because of the intrathecal water soluble contrast. The anterior and posterior rami (c) can be seen crossing the CSF to form the cervical nerve in the neural foramen (d)

The skull

Since the advent of CT, and more recently MRI, skull radiography has no role to play in the initial management of patients suspected of having structural intracranial pathology, as only the secondary effects of cerebral disease, e.g. evidence of raised intracranial pressure or calcification, are visible (Table 6.2).

Plain radiographs remain useful in abnormalities of the facial skeleton, in craniostenosis and in systemic disorders that may affect the bones of the face and skull, e.g. myeloma, hyperparathyroidism and haemoglobinopathies (Table 6.3).

Skull radiography is still performed in trauma patients when, in a fully orientated patient, there is a serious scalp laceration or haematoma, signs of a closed fracture or evidence of a foreign body or penetrating injury. These skull radiographs are always taken with a horizontal X-ray beam to enable fluid levels to be detected in the sinuses.

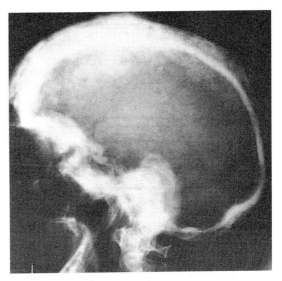

Figure 6.12 Paget's disease. Thickening of skull vault with ill-defined areas of sclerosis affecting both vault and base of skull. The neural foramina may be involved, leading to deafness

Table 6.2   Pathological intracranial calcification

Causes	Radiological features
● Vascular	
Atheroma	Curvilinear calcification, carotid syphon
Aneurysm	Related to main arteries
Angioma	Any site, both spotty and curvilinear
Sturge–Weber syndrome (rare). Clinically, a unilateral cutaneous facial haemangioma is present. Epileptiform convulsions occur	Tramline calcification – cortical
● Tumours	
Meningioma	Calcification in the tumour may be very dense. When related to sphenoid bone or vault, may produce localised sclerosis
Craniopharyngioma	Sella may be deformed. Calcification may be intra- or suprasellar. Such tumours in childhood are more frequently calcified than those occurring in adults
● Infection (rare)	
Tuberculosis	Involving the meninges, especially basal cisterns
Toxoplasmosis	May be paraventricular
Cytomegalic inclusion disease	Scattered foci
● Miscellaneous	
Hypoparathyroidism	Involving the basal ganglia
Tuberose sclerosis	Widely scattered foci of calcification

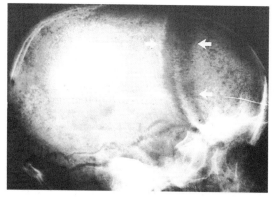

Figure 6.13   Small lytic secondary deposits in the skull vault from a neuroblastoma. Note apparent sutural diastasis due to parasutural deposits

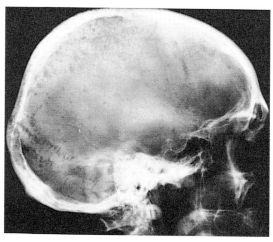

Figure 6.14   Small lytic lesions in the skull vault due to myelomatosis

Table 6.3 Abnormalities of the skull and facial bones

Causes	Radiological features
● Enlargement of skull vault	
Childhood	
hydrocephalus, raised intracranial pressure	Sutural diastasis, increased convolutional marking (i.e. 'copper beaten skull'). Bulging of fontanelle in infancy
Adults	
acromegaly	Enlarged frontal sinuses and mandible. Erosion and enlargement of sella turcica
Paget's disease	Thickened skull vault, increased density of vault and facial bones (Fig. 6.12)
● Increased density	
Localised	
hyperostosis frontalis interna	Common, especially in females. Symmetrical thickening of bone affecting inner table of vault. Of no clinical significance
meningioma	Area of localised sclerosis, may see enlarged vascular groove – due to the feeding artery
fibrous dysplasia	Asymmetrical. Affects facial bones, especially the maxilla, and base of the skull
Generalised	
Paget's disease	Irregular sclerosis with thickened vault (Fig. 6.12)
secondary deposits, e.g. prostate, breast	Multiple, ill-defined, small dense areas
osteopetrosis	Density affects skull vault and base – diffuse skeletal involvement
● Lytic lesions	
Childhood	
secondary deposits – neuroblastoma, leukaemia eosinophilic granuloma, (histiocytosis X)	Variable appearance – sutural deposit may mimic diastasis sutures (Fig. 6.13) Transradiant defect in vault, frquently edges are 'bevelled'
Adults	
myelomatosis	Rounded transradiancies, tend to be more sharply circumscribed than metastases, but frequently impossible to differentiate (Fig. 6.14)
secondary deposits	Generally multiple ill-defined transradiancies of varying size
hyperparathyroidism	Mottled appearance, classically 'pepper pot' skull
Paget's disease	Often associated with typical changes of Paget's disease elsewhere in the skeleton. Sharply defined transradiant zone, affecting large area of vault

Head injury

There is generally a poor correlation between the presence of a skull fracture on the plain radiograph and underlying brain damage, but when a fracture is detected the patient should be admitted for neurological observation (Table 6.4).

Any trauma patient who presents with neurological symptoms and signs should have a CT scan as the first investigation to detect any intracranial complications such as subdural and extradural haematomas (Fig. 6.16a,b), intracerebral haemorrhage, contusion, pneumocephalus, depressed or compound fractures and foreign bodies (Fig. 6.16c). CT can also be used to detect the secondary effects of trauma, such as oedema, ischaemia, infarction and hydrocephalus.

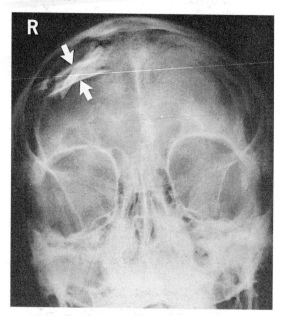

Figure 6.15a Depressed skull fracture – the degree of depression of the bony fragments can be seen in this example on the AP view. Frequently tangential views are necessary

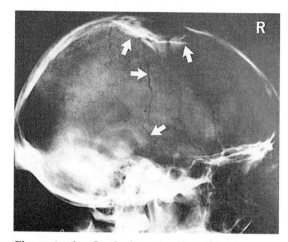

Figure 6.15b On the lateral radiograph a linear fracture is seen running through the temporo-parietal region, in addition to the depressed fragment. Compare the fracture line with the adjacent parallel vascular marking

Table 6.4 Skull fractures

Type of fracture	Radiological features
● Linear (Fig. 6.15)	Sharp transradiant line, may be straight or angled. May cross a vascular groove, e.g. that of the middle meningeal artery, or affect sinuses, e.g. frontal, and predispose to meningeal infection. Sutural diastasis may occur
● Depressed (Fig. 6.15)	May have curvilinear dense edges. More serious than a simple linear fracture. Tangential views are often necessary for the assessment of this type of fracture
● Base of skull	Difficult to detect radiologically. Suggested by the presence of a fluid level in the sphenoidal air sinus, cerebrospinal fluid rhinor-rhoea or bleeding from the ear

In the elderly, subdural haematomas can occur following relatively minor trauma. These patients deteriorate slowly, frequently becoming confused or developing localised neurological signs. Chronic subdural collections are of low density, have a characteristic shape and compress the underlying brain (Fig. 6.16d).

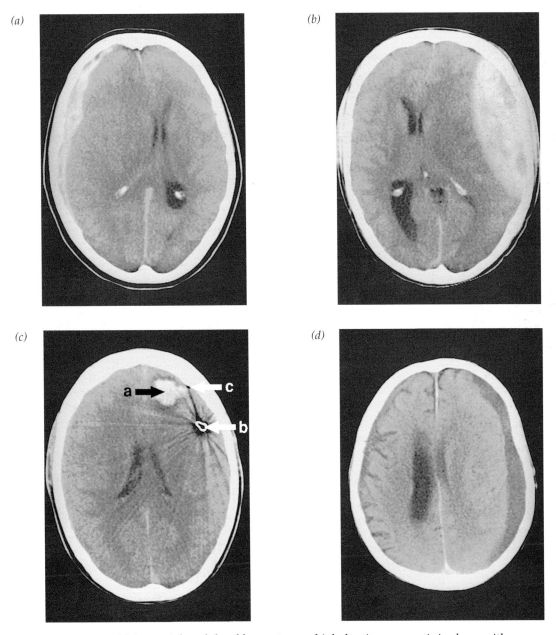

Figure 6.16 *(a)* Acute right subdural haematoma – high density, crescentic in shape with mass effect. Note the lateral ventricles are compressed and displaced. *(b)* Acute left extradural haematoma – lentiform in shape with mass effect. *(c)* Acute left frontal haematoma (a) following a gun shot injury. Artifact from bullet (b) and intracranial air (c). *(d)* Chronic left subdural haematoma-low density, crescentic in shape, and compressing the underlying sulci

(a)   *(b)*

(c)   *(d)*

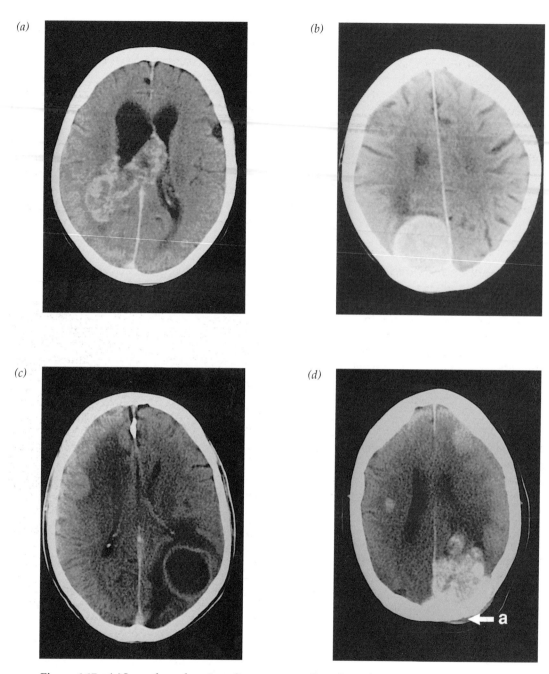

Figure 6.17   *(a)* Irregular enhancing glioma surrounding the right occipital horn and involving the corpus callosum. *(b)* Marked homogeneous enhancement of a convexity meningioma in the right posterior parietal region. *(c)* Right enhancement of a left posterior parietal brain abscess which is surrounded by oedema. Right frontal oedema associated with a second abscess is noted in this patient with subacute bacterial endocarditis (SBE). *(d)* Multiple enhancing metastases of varying sizes in a patient with known carcinoma of the lung. The bone in the left posterior parietal region is invaded and there is tumour extension into the subcutaneous soft tissues (a)

The brain

The introduction of MRI has revolutionised neuroradiological investigation. It is generally accepted as the investigation of choice for many neurological disorders. However, MRI is not yet widely available and many patients will still undergo CT. CT remains the investigation of choice for trauma and suspected intracranial haemorrhage, e.g. subarachnoid haemorrhage, which is of high density on CT.

Intracranial space-occupying lesions

Many may be suspected clinically in a patient who develops focal neurological signs or other evidence of raised intracranial pressure. CT, or when available MRI, should be carried out in these patients. Information is obtained to allow both diagnosis and the planning of appropriate treatment. No special patient preparation is needed before a CT or MRI head scan, either of which can be performed as an outpatient procedure. The head must be still during the scan to avoid motion artefacts, so patient co-operation is necessary. During CT a water-soluble contrast medium may be administered intravenously if a lesion is seen on the initial 'cuts'. If the lesion is vascular it tends to 'enhance' (increase in density), often in a characteristic fashion, e.g. a glioma will show irregular enhancement (Fig. 6.17a), meningiomas generally have a very marked homogeneous enhancement (Fig. 6.17b), and brain abscesses often have ring enhancement around the margins of the abscess (Fig. 6.17c). In addition, the scan can demonstrate the amount of associated cerebral oedema, the degree of midline shift and ventricular compression. Multiple mass lesions are most commonly due to cerebral metastases (Fig. 6.17d), but multiple abscesses can occur (Fig. 6.17c).

MRI is more sensitive than CT in detecting abnormalities within the brain. Magnetic resonance image quality is superior to CT, and images can be obtained in any plane. This can help the neurosurgeon to plan surgery. A paramagnetic contrast agent (gadolinium chelate) may be given intravenously to increase the sensitivity and conspicuity of lesions. When white matter pathology, e.g. demyelination (Fig. 6.18), temporal lobe epilepsy, lesions in the posterior fossa or meningeal disease are suspected clinically, MRI should be performed. As there is no signal from flowing blood, MRI is also helpful in the preoperative assessment of lesions adjacent to blood vessels. Magnetic resonance angiography (MRA) is a software option and allows images of the extracranial and intracranial blood vessels to be obtained non-invasively (Fig. 6.19).

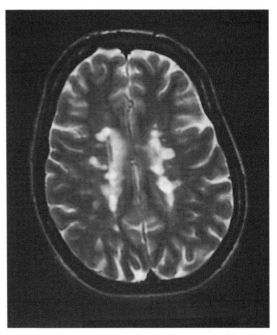

Figure 6.18 T2W axial MR brain scan. Multiple abnormal areas of increased signal are seen in a periventricular distribution and involving the corpus callosum in this patient with multiple sclerosis

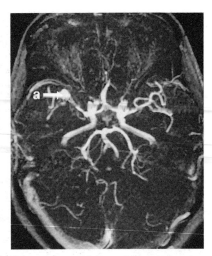

Figure 6.19   3D Time of Flight MRA showing the intracranial vessels. There is a right middle cerebral artery aneurysm present (a)

The ageing brain

A loss of cerebral tissue is part of the normal ageing process and is detected on CT. The cortical sulci and fissures enlarge with widening of the cerebrospinal fluid spaces overlying the brain and dilatation of the ventricular system (Fig. 6.20a). This dilatation must not be confused with hydrocephalus, which is a dilatation of the ventricular system resulting from an increase in the volume of cerebrospinal fluid due to a disturbance of its secretion, flow or absorption. In middle-aged or elderly patients atherosclerosis of the small intracerebral blood vessels, with or without accompanying hypertension, may result in multiple small areas of infarction in deep white and grey matter best seen on MRI (Fig. 6.20b). Patients with this picture may have signs of a multi-infarct dementia.

Cerebrovascular disease

Cerebral infarction may be suspected when a patient presents with an acute neurological deficit. This is commonly a result of ischaemia (embolic or thrombotic) (Fig. 6.20c), but a haematoma (Fig. 6.20d) needs to be differentiated by CT as there are management impli-

cations. Many patients who have a stroke will have an atherosclerotic plaque in the common carotid bifurcation and this can be non-invasively assessed by duplex ultrasonography or MRA.

Subarachnoid haemorrhage

The majority of cases are caused by rupture of an intracranial aneurysm. These are frequently small and located around the Circle of Willis. Less often bleeding is from an arteriovenous malformation or a rarer cause.

Clinically, patients with subarachnoid haemorrhage (SAH) have headache, neck stiffness, an altered level of consciousness, and/or neurological signs, e.g. a third nerve palsy due to pressure from a posterior communicating aneurysm. A lumbar puncture will reveal bloodstained cerebrospinal fluid after a SAH.

A CT scan in the early stages after a subarachnoid bleed will frequently show blood in subarachnoid, intracerebral or intraventricular locations (Fig. 6.21). Angiography is necessary to determine the exact site of the aneurysm and to see whether multiple aneurysms are present. If an arteriovenous malformation is present, its vascular supply and the draining vessels can be accurately shown by cerebral angiography.

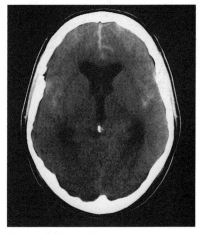

Figure 6.21   CT brain scan showing generalised subarachnoid blood and hydrocephalus, which is frequently seen soon after an acute SAH

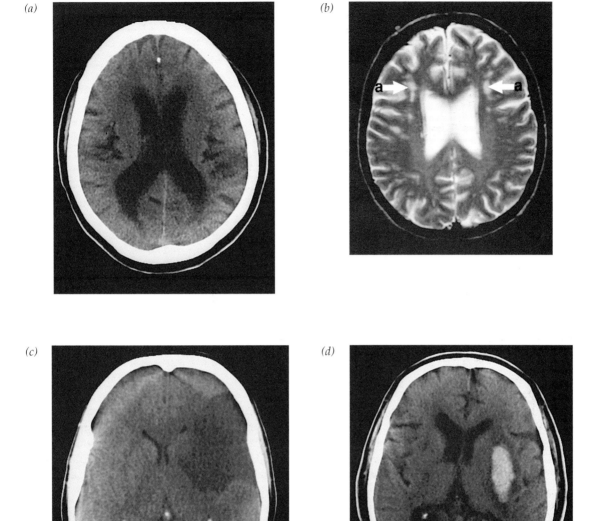

Figure 6.20 *(a)* CT brain scan showing cerebral atrophy. The ventricles are dilated. *(b)* T2W axial MR scan showing multiple areas of abnormal increased signal in the deep white matter (a), not in a periventricular distribution. These are areas of ischaemic damage/infarcts commonly seen in the older patient. *(c)* CT brain scan of an acute infarct in the left middle cerebral distribution. *(d)* CT brain scan of an acute left basal ganglia haematoma

Chapter 7

The breast; obstetric and paediatric radiology

The breast

- Mammography is complementary to clinical examination of the breast and is used predominantly to confirm or exclude the presence of cancer. Impalpable cancers may be demonstrated and preoperative localisation of such lesions is possible so that they may be biopsied.
- Mammography is also useful in the periodic assessment of the contralateral breast following mastectomy, and for monitoring the response of the cancer in the affected breast to non-surgical treatment.
- Breast ultrasonography can give further information, complementing clinical and mammographic assessment when there is a palpable mass or discrete mammographic lesion. It can differentiate between solid and cystic lesions and can be used to 'guide' biopsy needles.
- MRI is becoming established as a useful method for imaging breast disease, particularly where there has been previous treatment locally in the breast, in 'dense' breasts (where soft-tissue density is excessive and obscures lesions in mammography) or in making a full assessment of the extent of malignancy.
- In the UK National Breast Screening Programme asymptomatic women be-

tween the ages of 50 and 65 years are invited to undergo mammographic examination at 3 year intervals. Any suspicious lesions are assessed further by additional mammographic projections, clinical examination, ultrasonography and, when necessary, biopsy.

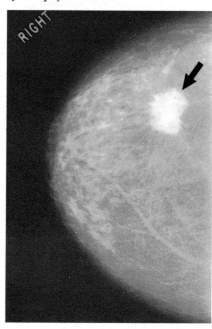

Figure 7.1 Film mammogram. Cranio-caudal projection showing a carcinoma in the breast – irregular spiculated mass (arrowed)

Mammographic features of breast cancer

The main fature of breast cancer is the presence of an irregular non-homogeous dense mass, which may be spiculated (Fig. 7.1). Microcalcifications (Fig. 7.2) are also a feature of malignancy. The overlying skin may be thickened and the nipple retracted; enlarged regional lymph nodes may be seen in those mammographic projections that include the axilla. A chest radiograph is indicated if more extensive involvement of the chest wall or more distant lymph nodes is suspected. Breast cancer is the most common cause of sclerotic bone metastases in women.

Benign lesions of the breast, on the other hand, are usually smooth in outline, have relatively low density and are homogenous (Fig. 7.3). Calcification, if present, is coarse (Fig. 7.4).

Ultrasonography in obstetrics

- Ultrasonography provides an accurate method of diagnosing pregnancy and its complications, and can be used to estimate the gestational age of the fetus. Fetal growth can be monitored and anomalies detected.
- In the very early stages of pregnancy transvaginal ultrasonography is more accurate than the abdominal technique and may detect the fetal heartbeat as early as 5 weeks gestation.
- Between 6 and 12 weeks fetal gestational age is calculated from the 'crown–rump' length. After this the biparietal diameter is used, along with other measurements such as the length of the femur or the circumference of the head or abdomen. Examples of images obtained at 18 weeks are shown in Figure 7.5.

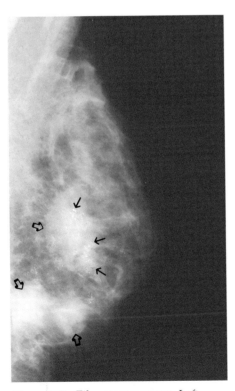

Figure 7.2 Film mammogram. Left oblique projection. Clusters of malignant micro-calcifications (arrowed) and three irregular densities representing invasive carcinomas (open arrows)

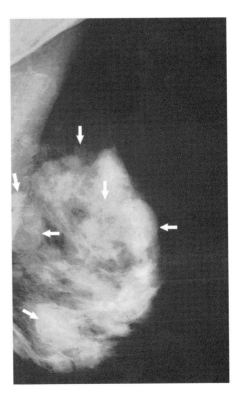

Figure 7.3 Film mammogram. Left oblique projection showing numerous cysts

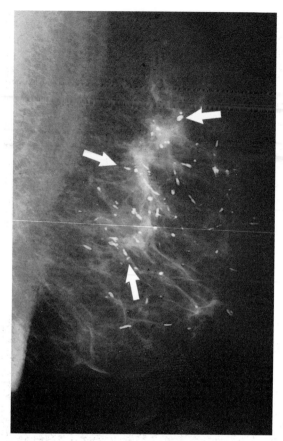

Figure 7.4 Film mammogram. Left oblique projection. Coarse calcification of benign disease scattered throughout the breast (arrows). Underlying pathology – plasma cell mastitis

- Multiple pregnancies can be detected using ultrasonography, as can a number of significant fetal abnormalities, including skeletal disorders such as spina bifida, renal abnormalities including cystic disease, and various abnormalities of the alimentary tract, e.g. exomphalos.
- The placenta can be assessed; this is important in cases of ante-partum haemorrhage and growth retardation. The position of the placenta is important when amniocentesis is to be performed and in cases of suspected placenta praevia late in pregnancy.

- Unsuspected pelvic disorders such as uterine fibroids or ovarian cysts may also be detected during routine obstetric ultra-sonography.

Paediatric radiology

This is an extensive field of sub-specialisation in diagnostic radiology and it is not the intention here to discuss paediatric problems and their radiological investigation in great detail.

In the paediatric age group there are quite well-defined combinations of clinical circumstances which lead to relatively intense periods of radiological investigation. Depending on their time of presentation these circumstances may be classified into four groups.

1. the fetus – problems detected during 'routine' or 'at risk' antenatal ultrasonography.
2. premature infants – several groups of disorders where an underlying disorder results in premature birth, or where the disorders encountered are attributable to the immaturity of the infant.
3. infancy – several significant congenital disorders may become apparent in early infancy; infants are also susceptible to some specific acquired disorders.
4. childhood – some congenital disorders present relatively late; alternatively those presenting in infancy may have long-term sequelae causing complications and ill health throughout childhood. Some of the acquired diseases in this age group require intensive radiological investigation.

The four groups are discussed in more detail in the following sections to demonstrate the role of imaging in the management of some of the disorders. It should be noted that there is some inevitable overlap between these four groups. A single disorder may be detected in the fetus, cause premature birth and cause complications throughout infancy and childhood.

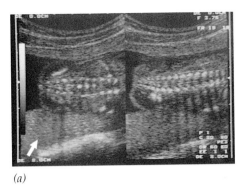

(a)

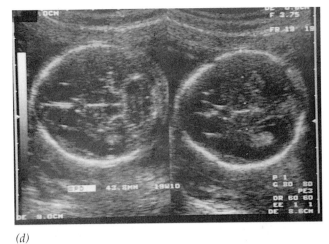

(d)

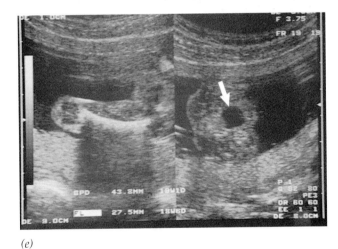

(e)

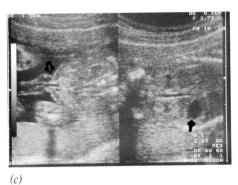

(b)

(c)

Figure 7.5   *(a)* and *(b)* Sagittal and longitudinal scans of the spine in an 18 week fetus. The placenta lies posteriorly (arrowed). *(c)* Views of the abdomen showing the umbilical cord insertion (open arrow) and the stomach (solid arrow). *(d)* Measuring the biparietal diameter. *(e)* Measuring the length of the femur to estimate gestational age. The bladder is visible on the adjacent scan (arrowed)

The fetus

Some disorders discovered at this stage are incompatible with life, e.g. some of the very severe dwarfing dysplasias, or severe cranial or spinal anomalies. Termination of pregnancy becomes an issue and the accuracy of the ultrasound information is crucial during the counselling process. If, on the other hand, the pregnancy runs its course, appropriate follow-up of the abnormality discovered during intrauterine life is carried out during the post-natal period. Examples include the following.

- *Growth disturbance*: non-lethal dysplasias of varying severity must be confirmed and classified using radiographic skeletal surveys. A full assessment of the skeleton is combined with clinical and genetic information to achieve an accurate diagnosis, which will in turn influence counselling of the parents and will enable the paediatricians and geneticists to assess the prognosis. This applies particularly to the management of severe or progressive skeletal deformities and their complications (Fig. 7.6).
- *Urinary tract problems*: dilatation of the urinary tract discovered 'in utero' may signify outflow obstruction (e.g. urethral valves in male infants), ureteric obstruction or vesicoureteric reflux. Post-natal

ultrasound examination and follow-up is necessary to assess the progression or regression of the dilatation. This may be combined with radionuclide imaging to assess both the degree of obstruction and renal function. Micturating cystourethrography is used to detect ureteric reflux and to define the anatomy of the bladder and urethra.

- *Alimentary tract disorders*: non-return of the embryonic gut into the abdominal cavity, in its varying forms, requires close monitoring during late pregnancy. These problems usually require surgical correction in infancy without the need for further radiological investigation. Where polyhydramnios is a problem in late pregnancy, an obstructing alimentary tract anomaly must be excluded. Causes include oesophageal atresia (Fig. 7.7) and other gut atresias and malformations. Plain chest and abdominal radiographs of the infant will give some indication of the site of obstruction (Fig. 7.8), although it takes several hours for swallowed air to reach the more distal parts of the intestinal tract. Therefore a sequence of abdominal radiographs may be necessary to demonstrate a distal obstruction. Clinical examination will detect anorectal anomalies. In cases of

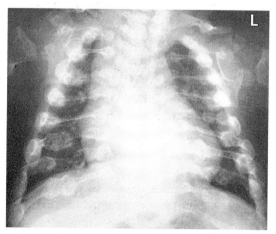

Figure 7.6　Numerous fractures in the thoracic cage of an infant with osteogenesis imperfecta

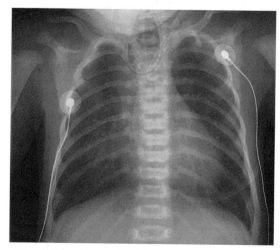

Figure 7.7　Infant with oesophageal atresia. Note the coiled nasogastric tube in the upper oesophagus

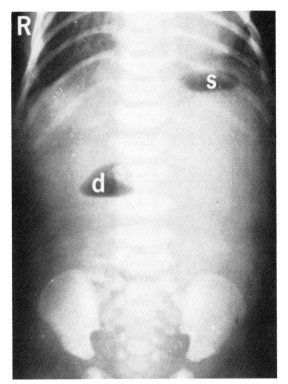

Figure 7.8 'Double-bubble' appearance on the erect radiograph of a neonate with Down's syndrome who has a duodenal atresia – note absence of air in remainder of small and large bowel

imperforate anus, inversion radiographs to show the distal point of the rectal atresia rarely affect the initial surgical management. Careful assessment of plain radiographs with clinical correlation usually determines whether surgical intervention is necessary. Contrast studies of the gut are rarely necessary and are contraindicated in suspected oesophageal atresia, where an opaque nasogastric tube usually demonstrates the obstruction quite adequately, as in Figure 7.7.

● *Skull or spinal disorders*: where pregnancy takes it full course and the infant survives, full neurological assessment will be followed by either ultrasonography of the brain, using the anterior fontanelle as a 'window', or CT. The latter is useful in cases of spiral dysraphism such as diastematomyelia.

Premature infants

Premature birth occurs relatively frequently when there are significant congenital disorders, but is itself associated with a pattern of complications where diagnostic imaging may play a significant part. Respiratory distress syndrome (RDS) due to surfactant deficiency causes typical lung abnormalities – diffuse fine nodularity and 'ground glass' appearance on a chest radiograph. The course of the disorder and its complications (which include pulmonary interstitial emphysema, pneumothorax, pneumomediastinum, and eventually bronchopulmonary dysplasia) can all be monitored radiographically. Intracranial bleeding, a well-recognised complication of prematurity, is detectable using trans-fontanellar ultrasound scanning. The progression of this disorder and the development of hydrocephalus and other serious brain complications can be monitored accurately.

Pseudo-obstruction of the alimentary tract may be due to 'immaturity' and abnormal motility, but this condition is difficult to distinguish from true organic obstruction due to bowel atresia, for example. Contrast studies of the gastrointestinal tract may become necessary for localisation of apparent obstruction and for determining the likely cause. The demonstration of an intact patent intestine allows a more conservative approach. Infants with prolonged bowel obstruction, whatever the underlying cause, are susceptible to necrotising enterocolitis (Fig. 7.9), which in turn may cause bowel perforation; bowel stricture is a late complication. In the acute phase, contrast studies of the bowel are absolutely contraindicated, but may be necessary for confirmation and localisation of stricture formation later.

Infancy

Table 7.1 summarises the radiological abnormalities seen in some of the common disorders of infancy that usually require radiological investigation. The table also indicates the variety of techniques that may be

Table 7.1   Common disorders of infancy

Causes	Radiological features [investigations]
● Respiratory distress	
RDS	Fine lung nodularity, variety of complications [CXR]
Meconium aspiration	Coarse nodularity, patchy consolidation and lung overinflation [CXR]
Infection	Patchy or lobar consolidation indistinguishable from aspiration [CXR, barium studies]
Congenital lung lesions	Cysts, sequestration. Characteristic sites usually [CXR]
Mass lesions	Paraspinal masses or cysts, e.g. neurenteric cyst; diaphragmatic hernia (Fig. 7.10) [CXR; ultrasonography; barium studies; CT]
Pulmonary oedema	Serious congenital heart disease [CXR; echocardiography; MRI; angiography]
● Growth disturbance and failure to thrive	
Skeletal dysplasias	Large variety, many having specific features [skeletal survey]
Alimentary disorders, malabsorption	Oesophageal reflux, malrotation, cystic fibrosis; bile-stained vomiting must be investigated [AXR; barium studies]
Failure to pass meconium	This is an early manifestation usually indicating a significant alimentary disorder, e.g. meconium ileus, unsuspected atresia or stenosis, aganglionic rectum or colon (Hirschsprung) [AXR; contrast studies – colon]
● Abdominal mass Site of origin is important – renal, suprarenal, hepatic	Early tumours, cystic kidneys, obstructed kidneys (hydronephrosis) – calcification is an important sign and occurs in neurogenic and liver tumours and in teratoma [AXR; ultrasonography; CT; contrast studies of the urinary tract; radionuclide imaging]

AXR, abdominal X-ray; CXR, chest X-ray.

necessary in the detection and management of these conditions. The list of disorders is illustrative and is not complete. Non-accidental skeletal trauma, for instance, is discussed in Chapter 5.

Childhood

Here a variety of acquired disorders such as chest infections, acute abdominal condi-tions (e.g. appendicitis), trauma and, less commonly, serious malignant disease such as leukaemia will require intensive radiological investigation. Chest radiographs, abdominal radiographs and ultrasonography, skeletal radiographs, and CT (and MRI) may be used respectively in the examples cited above. Those disorders that run prolonged and complicated courses require repeated investi-gations and radiological monitoring of

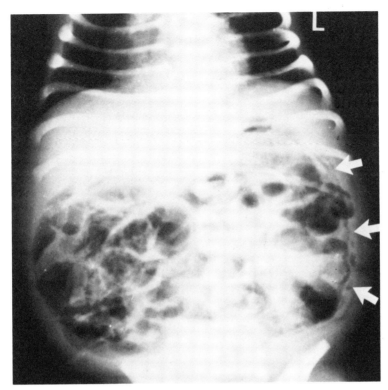

Figure 7.9   Gas in bowel wall of a neonate with necrotising enterocolitis – both linear and rounded transradiancies are evident, especially on the left side of the abdomen

(a)

(b)

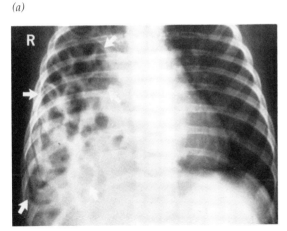

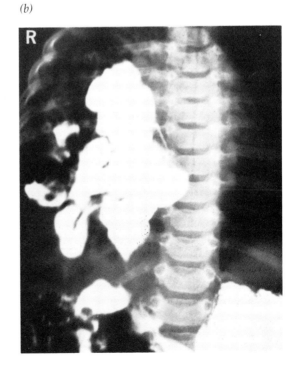

Figure 7.10   *(a)* Diaphragmatic hernia – 'cyst' like transradiant opacities seen in the right hemithorax. May occasionally be difficult to differentiate from a congenital cystic lung on plain radiographs. *(b)* Following administration of barium the intrathoracic small bowel loops are easily identified. This degree of bowel herniation is much commoner in left sided diaphragmatic defects. The underlying lung may be hypoplastic

response to treatment. If CT is the preferred modality then the child receives very significant doses of radiation; this must be balanced against the likely benefit and predicted clinical outcome.

Long-term sequelae of congenital disorders – neurological or cardiac anomalies, renal disease and cystic fibrosis for example – may necessitate repeated radiological investigation using plain radiographs and more complex techniques. Congenital heart disease may require angiography after initial assessment with echocardiography; MRI is playing an increasing role in this situation, allowing detailed non-invasive assessment of complex haemodynamic abnormalities due to congenital defects and shunts.

The course of cystic fibrosis is usually punctuated with acute episodes of chest infection (requiring repeated chest radiographs) and acute abdominal obstruction crises (such as meconium ileus equivalent and intussusception). The latter may necessitate ultrasound assessment or contrast studies. Portal hypertension due to liver fibrosis may justify contrast studies to assess the extent of oesophageal varices and the risk of bleeding. Consideration for heart/lung transplant requires extensive preparatory investigation using mainly CT.

Index